I0413378

THE REAL SKINNY ON FITNESS AND NUTRITION

Tips and Strategies from 13 Top Personal Trainers

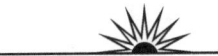

Compiled by:
Prominence Publishing
www.ProminencePublishing.com

Copyright © 2014 Prominence Publishing

All rights reserved.

ISBN-13:

978-1494472153

ISBN-10:

1494472155

Cover photo by
Crystal Allen of www.CrystalAllenPhotography.com

www.prominencepublishing.com

Disclaimer

This book is an educational product that provides general health information. The materials in The Real Skinny on Fitness and Nutrition: Tips and Strategies from 13 Top Personal Trainers are provided "as is" and without warranties of any kind either express or implied.

This book's content is not a substitute for direct, personal, professional medical care and diagnosis. None of the advice, diet plans, or exercises mentioned should be performed or otherwise used without clearance from your physician or health care provider. The information contained within is not intended to provide specific physical or mental health advice, or any other advice whatsoever, for any individual or company and should not be relied upon in that regard. We are not medical professionals and nothing in this book should be misconstrued to mean otherwise.

There may be risks associated with participating in activities mentioned in this book, for people in poor health or with pre-existing physical or mental health conditions. Because these risks exist, you should not participate in such diet plans if you are in poor health or have a pre-existing mental or physical condition. If you choose to follow any advice within this book, you do so of your own free will and accord, knowingly and voluntarily assuming all risks associated with such activities.

Facts and information are believed to be accurate at the time they were published in this book. All information provided is to be used for informational purposes only. Products and services described are only offered in jurisdictions where they may be legally offered. Information provided is not all-inclusive, and is limited to information that is made available. Such information should not be relied upon as all-inclusive or accurate.

You agree to hold SDI Communications, Prominence Publishing, its owners, agents, and employees harmless from any and all liability for all claims for damages due to injuries, including attorney fees and costs, incurred by you or caused to third parties by you, arising out of the fitness and diet plans discussed in this book.

Testimonials, case studies, and examples within this book are unverified results that have been forwarded to us by the interviewees featured in this book, and may not reflect the typical reader's experience, may not apply to the average person, and are not intended to represent or guarantee that anyone will achieve the same or similar results. You should always perform due diligence and not take such results at face value. We are not responsible for any errors or omissions in typical results information supplied to us by third parties.

TABLE OF CONTENTS

DEDICATION

This book is dedicated to the professional fitness experts who contributed their experience and wisdom, and to all their clients who have participated in their classes, groups and training sessions.

INTRODUCTION

If you've ever spent any amount of time browsing through the "Fitness & Nutrition" books section on Amazon or at your local book store, you've probably noticed one thing: There sure are a lot of books on the subject of losing weight and eating healthy. While this large amount of information on the subject may seem like a good thing, it could also be the one thing that keeps you from taking action towards your personal fitness and nutrition goals.

As you're probably aware, the fitness and nutrition industry is a multi-billion dollar industry. There are thousands upon thousands of people who rely on you to buy the next fitness book, exercise gadget, or DVD that hits the store shelves or the late night TV airwaves. Unfortunately, in this profit-driven world known as the fitness and nutrition industry, one priority gets lost: Getting <u>real results</u> for the client. You see, if one of these multi-million dollar companies actually produced a gadget or DVD that enabled everyone to be in the best shape of their lives forever, you wouldn't need to buy their products anymore—and that's exactly what they don't want to happen!

So what does this mean for you? Should you just throw in the towel and give up on any and all information out there? Of course not. You do, however, need to be more selective in where you get your information from.

The goal of this book was to interview highly qualified personal trainers who really train clients each and every day of their professional lives. Inside this book, you're not going to find interviews with celebrity fitness trainers. As you probably realize, most celebrity fitness trainers do very little day-to-day fitness training, because it conflicts with their schedules of book signings, producing DVDs, and filming television shows. It's sad to say, but many great personal trainers stop being great personal trainers the moment they get "discovered" by the "machine" that is the fitness and nutrition's marketing industry.

Consider this book to be the opposite of those glitzy, celebrity-endorsed books. When we produced this book, we set out to find real world experts and that's exactly what we got. Our biggest challenge was getting these personal trainers to break away from their busy schedules of training their clients, so that they could actually share their advice in this book. The trainers who have contributed to this book "walk the walk", and the content they've provided in the following chapters reflects their true knowledge and expertise. So, without further ado, we present to you, the real world expert interviews!

CHAPTER 1:

LIVE. TRAIN. EVOLVE.

Brian Washington started Live. Train. Evolve. in Malvern, PA, in 2008. Now a certified personal trainer with a degree in Sports Management, Brian still remembers how he started out. The facilities reflect a business that has been built from in-home personal training and fitness boot camps, using only the minimum of equipment to produce the desired results.

Live. Train. Evolve. is about a change in lifestyle, one that is tailored to the client.

What are some of the most common misconceptions that people have about hiring a personal trainer?

I often hear that it is too expensive to hire a personal trainer. When you are looking for a personal trainer, you should treat it like any other purchase you plan on making. Determine what you can afford to pay and look for the best prices for value, as higher rates do not always reflect how good a trainer is at their job.

What are some of the most common myths about nutrition?

When it comes to diet, everyone has different methods they believe work for them. Almost all of my clients say "I cut out carbs" or "I only eat 1-2 times a day". When I ask why, they respond with "because I am trying to lose weight". When it comes to diet and working out, I make each one of my clients understand that their nutrition is 80% of them being successful in reaching their fitness goals.

The amount of calories an individual consumes per day varies based on their caloric need. An average person should be eating about 4-6 meals a day, small and healthy meals. One thing that I say to my clients is "Eat clean and Eat often".

How soon, after someone starts a diet and exercise program, should they start to see results, to know if their diet and exercise program is working?

When someone starts a new exercise and diet program, the results will vary for each individual. One of the biggest things I tell my clients is that they can lose up to 1-2 lbs. per week safely. They can expect a change of anywhere from 4-8 lbs. per month.

What are some of the biggest mistakes that people make when they start an exercise program?

When I am completing a consultation I ask how many days per week they plan on working out. The answer is usually too high. People are anxious to lose weight and will start going 5-6 days a week. This is setting the individual up for failure. These individuals usually quit within 1-2 months or get stuck at a plateau.

Another mistake that I see is members doing the same routine every day. I tell the client to compare their first day in the gym to being in kindergarten. At first it will seem hard, but eventually you will get good at it, then you move on. If you stayed in kindergarten all your life of course you would be the best student, but you would never progress.

When you come in and lift the same weight and do the same movement you will become a pro at that action, but your results will be just as unchanging. Eventually it will be time to move on to a heavier weight or different movements. Most people get comfortable in the gym and are afraid to try new machines or new exercises.

Another mistake that I often see is women avoiding weights because of the myth of "getting bulky". This is a complete myth and women are missing out on the benefits of lifting weights including increased bone density, injury prevention, and a decrease in body fat.

How does someone know how hard to push themselves when they're working out?

Every exercise should be a challenge. If you are doing 3 sets of 10 on any exercise and you are not struggling on rep 9 or 10 then it's too easy; increase the weight. When it comes to cardio, if you can read while you are performing your cardio then it is too easy. Simply, you should be sweating.

If someone just recently had surgery, can they lift weights or work out? What should be taken into consideration in these situations?

Yes, they can lift and work out, but there are a few things that should be checked out first. Surgery is something that can hinder anyone's fitness goals. The first thing any experienced personal trainer should ask for is a doctor's note with any restrictions.

For example, if someone has had a recent hip replacement the doctor may give the individual a restriction of no hip flexion past 90 degrees. This would then rule out exercises such as squats. I have trained people post-surgery and each one has to be handled differently.

Is it possible to lose fat and gain muscle at the same time? If so, how can this be done effectively?

Yes, it is possible to lose to fat and gain muscle at that same time. This relates to nutrition and the basic formula of 3500 calories in one pound of fat. You need an adequate amount of calories to build muscle, and to burn fat you need a calorie deficit. For example, if someone is looking to lose weight but maintain muscle they will have to tap into stored calories.

Stored calories are in the body as fat. By cutting back on the amount of calories by 500 a day, in 7 days that person will cut out 3500 calories which equals to 1 pound of body fat.

With proper exercise and maintaining this calorie reduction over period of time, that person will cut body fat and increase muscle.

If someone has been a "yo-yo dieter" their entire life, how can a personal trainer help them?

The thing with a yo-yo diet is there is too much involved. With the common fad diets either you are cutting out foods that your body needs, or you have to buy foods in bulk and count points. That is too much to worry about in our busy lives. Personal trainers focus on showing the client how to continue to eat everyday foods by controlling the portion sizes and offering different ways of preparing their food.

With our consultation we give them a 7 day meal plan, showing them how they should be eating. We also give them the amount of calories they should be consuming, along with a grocery list and recipes. We have found this helpful because after the 7 days the person can begin to improvise or seek more help when needed. Instead of counting points they make healthy changes to their lifestyles, responsible only to themselves.

What is the difference between a "high impact" and a "low impact" workout?

High impact workouts involve exercises where both feet are leaving the ground, such as running, jumping, plyometrics, and cardio dance classes. These workouts are normally more intense and an individual can expect to burn more calories. High impact workouts also put individuals who have joint issues at higher risk for injury.

Lower impact workouts involve exercises where at least one foot remains on the ground. Lower impact exercises also decrease the amount of pounding and force on the joints. Water aerobics, cycling, and using the elliptical are all effective ways for clients with knee issues to get a cardio workout without the high impact stress of running.

How much of a say should the client have in determining which exercises they do?

We listen to the client and their body. A client knows what their body can handle and what it cannot. One thing that I say to each client is if there is an exercise you do not like let me know. There is always an alternate and we will find another way to work that same muscle. A client should have a say because my goal is to make their session enjoyable; not punishment.

Why do certain "non-fat" foods still make people gain weight?

Non-fat foods are altered versions of the original. When it comes to non-fat foods you have to first realize that the company removes certain ingredients and adds others to achieve the expected flavor, often by increasing sodium. Sodium has been shown to cause people to overeat.

Also, people believe the labels saying non-fat or low-fat to mean the food has fewer calories than the original and eat more of the altered food.

Is it true that some exercises produce results faster than others? Is so, which exercises provide the best and worst "returns on investment"?

One of the biggest complaints I hear from clients is how much and how long they have been running on the treadmill without losing any weight. Running on the treadmill is a bad investment, with repetitive movements and a chance of joint damage. When you run on a treadmill you do burn calories, but when you stop running you stop burning calories.

With resistance training you burn calories during and after your workout. The type of resistance training matters to how long you burn calories, but it can be 8-24 hours after you are done working out. Resistance training is the best investment for burning calories over time, but do not exclude cardio as part of your routine as it is important for heart health.

How should someone determine how many grams of protein and carbs they should be eating each day?

The USDA recommends anywhere from 1,000 to 3,200 calories. An individual will need to include other factors such as activity levels, weight loss goals, weight gain goals, and other health needs or restrictions. There are many different methods and formulas used to determine these results. One method that I use is BMR or Basal Metabolic Rate which is an estimate of how many calories your body burns daily.

Is it a good idea for someone to work out without a warm-up?

Never. Working out cold raises the risk of injury. The old school method was running or walking along with a static stretch to warm-up but this was shown to be ineffective. One of the methods being used now is dynamic warm-ups, which is a combination of stretching and cardio. Dynamic warm ups involved movements such as jumping jacks, lunges, high knee walking, and body weight squats.

Is it better to perform cardio before or after lifting weights, or should cardio be done on a completely different day?

If you are going to do cardio on the same day you are lifting I prefer the cardio to be done after. You will need the energy for lifting weights, making your workout safer. It also allows you to give your weight training 100% and use your cardio as a finisher. This will also make your cardio session seem that much harder.

I would recommend doing your cardio on your off days, when you aren't lifting weights. This is called active rest as you are still active but using different muscles, letting the muscles used for lifting rest.

Is it better to exercise every part of the body on the same day, or is it better to focus on different muscle groups on different days?

This all depends on what the person is training for. Functional training uses exercises that replicate everyday movements such as squatting and lifting your kids or groceries. This is different than training for a marathon or particular sport. Someone who is looking to body build or show bigger muscle gains should focus on particular parts such as back and biceps or chest and triceps.

I would recommend a total body circuit workout. This is because in your everyday life you usually do all of these movements back to back, such as push and pulling or lifting and twisting. Exercising using the same muscles will help you do those everyday activities without injury, such as throwing out your back.

If someone doesn't have the time to spend hours cooking healthy meals, how can they still eat healthy?

Make the time to prepare and pack your meals. The best thing to do is prepare your meals for the week a few days before hand. Another thing that I offer my clients is options they can get when they are out and about. For example, taking the kids to a fast food restaurant and you are hungry too. Sometimes that salad option with the special dressing is not the healthiest. The grilled chicken sandwich, plain with veggies, may be the better option but that depends on the restaurant. Educating yourself on certain menu options at restaurants will carry you a long way.

What should a personal trainer take into consideration when working with each individual client?

What I focus on is medical history, realistic goals, and time frame. I really want to be honest with every client and I want them to have realistic goals. When they know what to expect this will increase their success rate and their overall happiness. I also take all of this information into account when developing their workout plans and diets. If they have restrictions such as joint pain or allergies to certain foods I can alter their plans so that we can progress at the right pace.

If someone isn't sore after a workout, does that mean they didn't work out hard enough?

You should expect soreness after your first few workouts. This soreness is DOMS, or Delay Onset Muscle Soreness. Over time your soreness will decrease as your body becomes used to working-out. If DOMS does not decrease over time, you may need to adjust your workout. You might not be resting adequately between workouts or you may be pushing your physical limits, or even damaging your body. Soreness after a workout is not a good or accurate gauge of how effective the workout was.

The new fad seems to be "buying organic". Is there any validity to eating organic food over non-organic food? What are the benefits and/ or things to be aware of?

Buying organic is a personal preference. Organic foods are usually free of pesticides and any additional hormones used to increase the growth process of the food item. Organic foods are normally higher in price than the non-organic brand. Organic foods have not been proven to give anyone a higher fitness advantage but if you want to avoid putting certain pesticides and chemicals in your body than organic is the way to go.

—

Brian Washington, Owner
Live. Train. Evolve.
147 W King St Unit C
Malvern, PA 19355
484-927-6177 brian@livetrainevolve.com
www.livetrainevolve.com

At Live. Train. Evolve. we offer affordable personal training, boot camps, kickboxing, and sports performance training. Unlike your average big box gym we offer personalized fitness services. Whether you are a beginner or a seasoned athlete, we are trained to handle all skill levels and help you reach your goals.

CHAPTER 2:

BODYSMITH GYM & STUDIOS

Established in 1998, BodySmith Gym & Studios has a state-of-the-art gym, complete with an organic shake and juice bar. For those dazzled by the array of machines, personal trainers have their own area to help that client achieve their goals. A wide variety of classes, boot camps, and other activities are sure to help anyone find a physical activity they can enjoy.

How soon after someone starts a diet and exercise program should they start to see results, to know if their diet and exercise program is working?

The first thing everyone must understand is that each individual is different, with different goals and different physical capabilities. We believe that each person should take a realistic approach to health to complement their lifestyle. Creating realistic goals and habits will make any goal achievable and sustainable. With that being said, all clients should start to notice a difference within week 1.

The body can change quickly if all of the elements (diet, cardio, and resistance training) are incorporated. The initial changes may only be neuromuscular but these changes will help facilitate the ultimate goals of weight loss or muscle growth in the future. The real changes with weight loss and muscle gains can take weeks to see depending on factors including recovery (sleep and diet).

What are some of the most common misconceptions that people have about hiring a personal trainer?

Many clients think that hiring a personal trainer is a magic solution for achieving their goals. Personal Training will offer guidance, accountability, and a specialized program geared towards the individual, but the real work lies with the client themselves. Diet, cardio, and sleep play very important roles to success.

What are some of the most common myths about nutrition?

We can talk for days about common myths about nutrition. Perhaps a large misconception is that eating healthy foods will help you lose weight no matter what. I have many clients that eat salads without examining the amount of calories being consumed. While the salad may be healthy, portion size and toppings make a big difference. A 2000 calorie salad won't help you to lose weight. Portion control and calorie expenditure play a large role in success. Eat your salad but watch your toppings and portions.

What are some of the biggest mistakes that people make when they start an exercise program?

I believe there are two big mistakes people make when they start an exercise program.

1) Many people create unrealistic goals and don't allow for proper progression within a program. I have clients that haven't exercised in years and think they are ready to weight train 5 days per week. Matching your goals with your lifestyle will make your program more successful in the long run. Along with your goals, your program may have to consider other factors like injuries or imbalances that you've accrued over the years. Making sure your body is well aligned and injury free will make your workouts more efficient and promote long term success.

2) Each workout doesn't have to take 120% as long as you are progressing safely toward your goals. Proper progression will ensure a

successful workout every time and won't debilitate you for a whole week. This is about long-term success and being realistic with your goals.

How does someone know how hard to push themselves when they're working out?

Factors like current fitness level, injuries, sleep, and diet all play a large role in how hard a person can push themselves when working out. Even with advanced athletes there is a time to back off high intensity workouts. Most clients don't fall in the category of having to worry about overtraining but it's something to consider.

If you are just starting out on a program, form takes the front seat and intensity comes later. A program should have a systematic approach that allows for successful lifts with good form, teaching you to do the movement without injury.

If someone just recently had surgery, can they lift weights or workout? What should be taken into consideration in these situations?

As with any medical issue a doctor should have the final say in whether a client is ready to lift weights. I don't think there's a trainer out there that should make that decision.

Is it possible to lose fat and gain muscle at the same time? If so, how can this be done effectively?

It is possible to lose fat and gain muscle at the same time with a well-rounded approach, incorporating a great diet, good recovery, and a resistance training program of at least 3 days per week. Having a goal like this needs patience and a well tracked program. Keep your eye on the long term goal and you can succeed!

If someone has been a "yo-yo dieter" their entire lives, how can a personal trainer help people like this?

I believe any great trainer can help a client to create consistency in their daily life. "Yo-yo dieters" need a realistic approach to nutrition and accountability to stay on target. A personal trainer can offer this to a client by checking in, setting goals, and assessing to make sure the client stays on track.

What is the difference between a "high impact" and a "low impact" workout?

A "high impact" workout generally involves plyometrics, jumping, running, and/or explosive movements. The term "high impact" usually describes how your joints absorb the movement and is generally used in circuit, sport specific, and explosive training. Plyo box jumps are high impact. "Low-impact" would be the opposite but doesn't necessarily mean low weight. Typically clients with major issues in their knees or low back should avoid high impact training as it can be hard on the joints.

How much of a say should the client have in determining which exercises they do?

Generally I feel like the trainer should be directing the workout and this includes exercise selection. It is important for the trainer, however, to listen to the client and make the best decision for their success. If a client is uncomfortable with a movement or feels pain, it might be a smart decision to change exercises.

I'm a firm believer that a client should feel like they're going in the right direction and sometimes giving them some control in exercise selection can be helpful.

Why do certain "non-fat" foods still make people gain weight?

Calories in vs. calories out are what determine if you gain or lose weight. While controlling your total calories is important, the nutritional value of those calories is equally important. Many people don't realize that eaten "fat" is not what makes up stored body fat. "Non-fat" foods that contain sugar can be stored as fat in the body when the body doesn't use it as energy. Wine is a common culprit for gaining weight and it's because of sugar . . . not fat.

Is it true that some exercises produce results faster than others? Is so, which exercises provide the best and worst "returns on investment"?

No matter if you want to lose weight or gain muscle, larger muscle groups have the biggest impact on your entire body. If increasing muscle mass or increasing your resting metabolic rate is your goal, then larger muscles should be trained. Why would I train biceps (a small muscle group) if I want to increase muscle mass or my resting metabolic rate? Compound movements for legs and back are the secret to losing weight or gaining muscle. They will affect your entire body. With that being said, deadlifts, squats and any pulling movements are my favorites for success.

How should someone determine how many grams of protein and carbs they should be eating each day?

Genetics, age, weight, fitness level and goals all play a role in determining how many grams of protein or carbs to consume each day. More advanced athletes can consume close to 2 grams of protein per pound of bodyweight. Typically, individuals should fall between .5 and 1 grams of protein per pound of bodyweight.

Carbs can be trickier, depending on goals and the types of carbs. Carbs are everyone's primary source of energy and therefore should be consumed in larger amounts, but different types are needed in different amounts. Complex carbohydrates should take priorities over simple sugars, especially when trying to lose weight.

Is it a good idea for someone to workout if they have a cold?

The saying typically goes, "If the cold is neck up then you're safe to workout. If the cold is neck down (in your chest) you should probably lay off." An intense workout can certainly lower your immune system for a short time so always err on the side of caution. Workout intensities and fitness levels also play a role in how the workout will affect you.

Is it better to perform cardio before or after lifting weights or should cardio be done on a completely different day?

If your goal is to lose weight then I would suggest adding 15 minutes of cardio to the end of each weight lifting session. Additional cardio sessions are suggested on days without weight lifting as well. On the days that cardio is done by itself (with weight loss goals) clients should focus on the duration first and the intensity second. Build up to a 45-60 minute workout and then gradually increase the intensity. For muscle mass goals, less cardio is required.

Is it better to exercise every part of the body on the same day, or it better to focus on different muscle groups on different days?

Ultimately the individual's goals, fitness level, and training days per week answer this question. If a client is only weight training 2 times per week then a full body workout is more important. If a client is training 3 or more days per week then it becomes more important to train different body parts each day. The main goal with weight training is to build strength and muscle.

Getting a client to a point where they're training more days per week is best for a client's success. With this scenario clients can have more focused workouts per body part and subsequently will get stronger and build muscle faster.

If someone doesn't have the time to spend hours cooking healthy meals, how can they still eat healthy?

Cooking your own meals is the best way to ensure healthy choices.

What should a personal trainer take into consideration when working with each individual client?

Success for each individual can come in many forms. The most important thing for a trainer to consider with each client is what determines their success. It's important not to downplay small advances for each person as the small successes can lead to big things. I've trained advanced athletes that love to train, listen to everything I say, and make quick progress achieving their goals. What is most rewarding for me is the client with more challenges. To me, success is if I can get someone who hates exercise to work out and follow healthy guidelines. Even making the smallest changes in an unhealthy lifestyle can be the small step that leads to great things!

If someone isn't sore after a workout, does that mean they didn't work out hard enough?

It's not important to be sore after every workout. Workout intensities should vary and therefore soreness should vary as well. I'll go a step further to say that you should never have soreness that's debilitating. A great trainer can have you feel a workout but wanting more, and proper progression is key.

The new fad seems to be "buying organic". Is there any validity to eating organic food over non-organic food? What are the benefits and/ or things to be aware of?

There's little regulation on "organic" VS "non-organic" food. I don't think there's enough research to say "organic" food is more nutritious or less harmful than conventional foods.

—

Shane Beatty, General Manager/Trainer
BodySmith Gym & Studios
1630 14th St NW,
Washington DC 20009
Shane Beatty
202-468-0858

Shane@bodysmithgym.com
Www.bodysmithgym.com

Shane Beatty and BodySmith Gym & Studios have been the pioneers in the training business since 1998. We offer a personal approach to fitness. We are a true neighborhood gym and clients feel when they walk through our doors that everyone is welcome!

CHAPTER 3:

JESSICA MANNING

PERSONAL TRAINING

Jessica Manning uses her expertise to show clients the difference between fad diets and real, sustainable changes to their lifestyle. With a positive attitude and the right knowledge, clients are given the chance to lead better, more balanced, lives.

How does someone tone up and lose fat under their arms and around their triceps?

To lose fat, you cannot spot tone. You must strength train every muscle in the body for proper muscle tone, but strength training also leads to an increased metabolism, which results in fat loss. Adequate cardiovascular exercise, clean and balanced nutrition, and strength training will turn you into a well-oiled fat burning machine. Exercises like Overhead Triceps Extensions and Triceps Dips will improve definition and strengthen the triceps.

For people who are always tired, won't working out make them feel like they have even less energy?

Chronic fatigue or lethargy often comes from a lack of exercise and a sluggish metabolism. Assuming energy loss is not from having simply lost too much sleep or being overworked, exercise will help to pump blood through the body, oxygenating and regenerating the cells. It will result in having more energy and being more mentally alert.

What's the difference between "good carbs" and "bad carbs"?

This answer doesn't just apply to carbs, but to all food groups: "Good" foods provide a lot of nutritional bang for buck (deliver a lot of nutrition for the calories / energy content), and "bad" foods contain very little nutritional value for the calories. We call these "bad" foods empty calories. Carbs that are highly processed and refined typically provide few natural nutrients, and instead provide chemicals and preservatives.

Try to stick to vegetables, fruits, whole grains, legumes . . . foods that are the most natural and come right out of the ground.

Is it true that stress makes people gain weight? What is the truth, if any, behind this?

Stress triggers a hormone called cortisol which promotes fat storage in the abdominal region. Not only does it cause fat gain because of its hormonal consequences, but stress also has us reaching for foods that are quick fixes like simple carbohydrates and sugars. These foods temporarily suppress stress by releasing serotonin, a feel-good chemical in the brain. This feeling is very short-lived because these foods also trigger addiction, which brings a lack of control, which spurs stress levels.

Look for healthier ways to de-stress, such as exercising, cooking healthy meals, and conversations with friends and family.

Fish seems to have a lot of fat in it. Will people gain weight if they eat too much fish?

Fish contains a healthier fat than that found in land animals. Healthy fats are very good for the body and contribute to a healthy metabolism, which helps in losing excess fat from our bodies. Consuming fish 2-3 times a week is recommended for most people.

Besides fish, look for other healthy sources of fat, such as nuts, avocados, and olives.

If someone is a heavy smoker, should their workout routine be adjusted at all? If so, how?

Heavy smokers can probably expect a quicker and steeper increase in their heart rate during exercise, because of the corruption to the arteries. Smokers tend to have high blood pressure, meaning the heart has to work harder to push blood through the arteries (likely because of toxic blockages), and therefore need to perform at a slightly lower intensity. Your best bet is to quit smoking as the risks of smoking begin to decrease right away. Soon you will enjoy a much improved fitness level and be able to exert yourself without such cardiovascular obstacles.

Is there any truth to the claim that exercise can help improve brain function and/or mental focus? If yes, how?

Exercise requires mental focus, as we require our brains to trigger certain muscles and to control our breathing. Exercise also slows the aging process, and this includes the brain. The body's natural decaying process is prolonged with physical activity, and the brain is a part of the body!

When people say they need to run to "clear their head", there is truth to this. Focusing on a specific task while physically expelling one's negative energies, such as stress or frustration, help us to remove mental obstacles and therefore be more alert to our needs.

What are the biggest mistakes people make when hiring a personal trainer?

Investing the money before they are really ready to work is a common mistake. A personal trainer's job is to push you out of your comfort zone, provide you with efficient challenges, and help you to make positive changes to your diet. A personal trainer is not a gadget on an infomercial that you can just purchase on a whim, when you are not ready to make a change.

If you want a trainer to emotionally invest in helping you to make positive life changes, you must make that same mental commitment. It can be the best investment you've ever made, or it can be a ton of money lost. Wasting your time and money will only lead to discouragement, for you and the trainer who wanted to help you be your best self.

What can people do to avoid back injuries when they're lifting weights?

Train and engage the core muscles, with mental focus on doing the exercises correctly. A proper core program will include isolated abdominal training, isolated lower back training, exercises that combine the two (like the plank), as well as compound stability exercises (such as a squat on a BOSU ball).

Assuming you are including core exercises into your program, keep your core taut while executing other moves like dead lifts, squats, lat pull-down, etc. You will learn to engage your core by thinking about it, and therefore be protecting your lower back with strength in the abdominals during all aspects of your workout.

If someone eats very healthy, and they have an active lifestyle, do they still need to work out? Why or why not?

Everybody should have a specifically catered strength program because it helps to balance out their anatomy. Every single body has quirks that build up over time (a cranky knee from running, a tight hip flexor from driving too much, a weakened upper back from working at a computer). It is important to train in order to correct these imbalances before they begin to affect the skeletal system, which can then lead to a susceptibility to injuries and uncomfortable aging.

Strength training exercises are necessary for preventing/improving arthritis and other joint pain. We should pay attention to and strengthen every part of our bodies, in order for them to be able to do more for us, longer.

Do minors typically need to get the permission of an adult or guardian if they want to work with a personal trainer? If so, how does this work?

All minors need permission from an adult before beginning a fitness program with a trainer. Most trainers are (and should be) insured, but some are not insured to work with minors. Only trainers who are insured to work with minors may do so.

Minors and their parents should receive verification that their trainer is skilled with functional movements related to still growing bodies. Children should not be lifting heavy, if any, weights—just doing body weight movements.

Why do some people lift heavy weights while other people lift lighter amounts of weights?

Some people lift heavy weights and others lift lighter ones because they have probably been told that is best for their specific goals. Women often hear that lighter weights will result in smaller muscles, and men often believe that lifting heavier is better for bulk. In truth, everyone should lift to their best of their abilities, without sacrificing form. For example, men who feel better about curling 50 lbs. dumbbells for their biceps may be swinging their arms back in order to lift the weight, which is not beneficial for strengthening the bicep in isolation.

Most women do not have the testosterone to build bulky muscles, and so they need not be concerned that they will become too "big". Both men and women should change things up occasionally by doing what is called periodization training; spending 6 weeks doing lighter weights fatiguing between 15-20 reps, 6 weeks fatiguing between 8-12 reps, and 6 weeks fatiguing between 4-8 reps.

Do personal trainers normally work with clients who are only free on weekends or during off-hours? What's typical in terms of when personal trainers are available?

It is up to individual trainers to make their own schedules. I take weekends off, because I accommodate clients from early morning to early afternoon, and then from late afternoon to late evening.

In order to remain passionate and energized to inspire and teach people, I must remain balanced in my own life. I need time for rest, my own workouts, and friends and family just like those who work a 9-5 Monday to Friday workweek. A career is a career, and we all must achieve balance to stay great at our jobs!

If someone has back problems, or other physical limitations, how can they lift weights safely, without getting hurt?

A qualified trainer will know what adjustments to make to each exercise and with each physical limitation will be necessary for people with back problems. If you do not have the knowledge yourself about how to proceed, you are at risk of making the injury worse.

What is the typical way to pay a personal trainer? Weekly? Monthly? At each session?

This is the trainer's decision coming from how he/she makes a living and runs a business. More often than not, sessions are sold in lump sums, and then the trainer and the client decide together how the sessions will be spaced out. Clients renew on their last paid session, so that each session is paid in advance to protect the trainer should the client cancel last minute (which may come with a default penalty).

When is a spotter needed for exercises?

When an exerciser is training to failure (recommended for best results), it is imperative to have a spotter to prevent the exerciser from losing control of the weights. A spotter can jump in when the muscle fails or nearly fails to complete a repetition, before gravity pulls on the weight and there is risk of injury. When gravity pulls on the weight and the muscle has lost control, the muscle becomes very vulnerable to being torn—or worse, injured so severely that it affects the joint.

How does someone tone up in specific "problem areas"?

You cannot spot tone, i.e. remove body fat from one area, but you can use isolated movements to further shape one muscle group. The best shaping, however, is done with strengthening alongside losing fat, and so these 3 factors are of equal importance: clean eating, cardiovascular activity, and strengthening exercises. All three of these components results in a lean, fit, healthy and energized physique with toned assets.

Is it true that too much cardio can be unhealthy?

Too much cardio results in burning muscle, overusing the heart, and negatively impacting the joints. There needs to be a balance of strength training and cardio, with adequate fuel (food) in order to keep the metabolism spiked and the joints sustainably healthy.

What are the benefits of hiring a personal trainer over just buying some DVDs that feature personal trainers?

Hiring a personal trainer guarantees that you will be equipped with a program or a way of exercising that is specifically catered to your strengths and weaknesses, likes and dislikes (which are imperative for staying motivated and performing your best) and for form correction. Tiny changes to the form of an exercise can make a world of difference in the results that you achieve, as well as the injuries you avoid.

Is it a good idea to walk or run with weights? Will this produce results more quickly?

It can burn more calories, yes, like how a heavier person burns more calories because they have more of a challenge to move around. So, adding weights makes you heavier, and therefore you can burn more calories. But, carrying weights will disrupt the natural rhythm of the exercise, of walking or running, and I believe in keeping it simple. General exercise is for a healthy heart, high energy, and endurance. Strength train for an increased metabolism, a tight and lean physique, and eat clean for nutritional density—to keep the good and lose the excess fat.

—

Jessica Manning, Owner/Personal Trainer
Pure Transformation Personal Training
Toronto Ontario
647-881-5479
www.JessicaManning.com
www.PureTransformation.ca

This company filters the confusion in the fitness/wellness industry. We provide a strong emphasis on correct form, on creative and functional movements, and on balanced and clean eating. All of our methods are sustainable for life, and therefore lead to permanent results.

CHAPTER 4:

TRAIN WITH LISA

Lisa Boucher offers in-home personal training for most of Utah County. Certified in personal training and fitness instruction, Lisa also authored a sugar free cookbook and supplies healthy, unprocessed nuts from her website. Her belief in a healthy, nutritious, balanced lifestyle is a part of everyday life for her family and she can make it part of her client's lives as well.

For people who are always tired, won't working out make them feel like they have even less energy?

Exercise actually increases energy and can help fight fatigue. Although it may seem like exercise does the opposite, studies show that those who work out regularly are stronger, have more energy, and experience better moods.

How does someone tone up and lose fat under their arms and around their triceps?

There is no such thing as "spot reducing". You can "tone up" as much as you want by picking specific exercises that target problem areas but you will never see any of the results from your hard work if it is covered with a layer of fat.

In order to lose fat you have to burn more calories than you are consuming. One of the best ways to do this is cardio, specifically, interval training.

What's the difference between "good carbs" and "bad carbs"?

"Good Carbs" refer to complex carbohydrates and "bad carbs" refer to simple carbohydrates. Simple carbs are foods with a chemical structure that is composed of 1 or 2 sugars. They are refined sugars that have very little nutritional value.

Complex carbs have a chemical structure that is made up of 3 or more sugars which are usually linked together to form a chain. These sugars are rich in fiber, vitamins, and minerals. These foods, because they are complex, take longer to digest, which provides the body greater satiation. These complex or "good" carbs are the carbs we should be consuming.

Is it true that stress makes people gain weight? What is the truth, if any, behind this?

It is absolutely true that stress can cause weight gain. On a physiological level: when we experience stress, the body releases hormones, including cortisol. Elevated levels of cortisol can lead to an increase in appetite, which then leads to over consumption of food.

On an emotional level, when stressed, people look to food as an immediate source of comfort. And it's not usually healthy fare—it's more of the comfort foods—think fatty, sweet, calorie dense etc.

Fish seems to have a lot of fat in it. Will people gain weight if they eat too much fish?

There are good fats and bad fats. Fish have Omega-3 fatty acids, the good fat. Our bodies need Omega-3's. Fish should be part of your healthy diet. However, if you are preparing your fish in a lot of butters, oils, and batter, your fish will make you gain weight. If you are not a fish lover you can ensure your Omega-3 consumption by taking a reputable fish oil supplement.

If someone is a heavy smoker, should their workout routine be adjusted at all? If so, how?

Smoking never has been, nor will it ever be, part of a healthy lifestyle. However, if you smoke and exercise you will need to adjust the intensity of the exercise to fit your capabilities, as your training endurance will be reduced. For a smoker, the heart will have to work even harder for oxygen to reach your tissues—this means that the heart will have to beat faster in exercise for a smoker than a non-smoker.

Is there any truth to the claim that exercise can help improve brain function and/or mental focus? If yes, how?

Exercise increases oxygen flow to the brain and can, over time, reduce the risk of disorders that lead to memory loss. In addition to that benefit, the increased oxygen can immediately improve focus and productivity.

What are the biggest mistakes people make when hiring a personal trainer?

They hire a personal trainer without researching and base their decision on price. Just because the price is right, doesn't mean the trainer is. Make sure the trainer is certified, experienced, and can work with your specific concerns. Be honest and open with your trainer. A trainer can only help you as much as you let him/her. Tell your trainer about past injuries, present physical concerns, diet issues etc. so that your trainer can work for you.

A qualified trainer will keep you safe while guiding you through fantastic workouts. Don't expect your trainer to work miracles though—the hard work comes from you. If you don't follow through with your trainer's expectations, you will not see results.

What can people do to avoid back injuries when they're lifting weights?

A great trainer will always incorporate core work, and even more so if you suffer from back injuries because a stronger core means a stronger back. However, a trainer cannot feel your pain so you have to be extremely communicative with him/her to let them know your limitations. If you cannot lift weights with perfect form, chances are your weight is too high for you. Always pick a weight that is challenging but allows you to maintain great form. Never sacrifice form for higher weight; that is how injuries happen.

If someone eats very healthy, and they have an active lifestyle, do they still need to work out? Why or why not?

Eating a healthful diet is necessary for good nutrition. Exercise is necessary for optimal physical strength and endurance. The two together are the perfect combination for a healthy lifestyle. One cannot replace the other. Even if you eat well, you still have to exercise.

Do minors typically need to get the permission of an adult or guardian, if they want to work with a personal trainer? If so, how does this work?

Minors need the permission of their legal guardian in order to participate in a personal training program. Many trainers require a signed form, as well as a doctor's note regarding the individual's health, before the minor can begin.

Why do some people lift heavy weights while other people lift lighter amounts of weights?

Typically, people who lift heavy weights have different goals than those who lift lighter weights. Heavier weights are used for building muscle mass or size, while lighter weights are used for tightening and toning.

However, many gym goers (specifically women) need to rethink what they consider "light". They tend to lift lighter because they fear getting too bulky. Don't worry ladies; we don't have enough testosterone to bulk up like a man. Lift weights that are heavy enough that you reach failure within 12-15 reps.

Do personal trainers normally work with clients who are only free on weekends or during off-hours? What's typical in terms of when personal trainers are available?

Personal training is exactly what the name implies: personal. All trainers are different and offer different hours for their clients. Most gyms offer personal trainers that work days, evenings, and weekends. Self-employed trainers set their own schedule.

If someone has back problems, or other physical limitations, how can they lift weights safely, without getting hurt?

Proper form is everything when it comes to safety. A good, qualified trainer will always emphasize proper form through any exercise. When someone does have back problems, typically they have certain guidelines from their doctor, which will include exercises they should and should not do. Share these limitations with your trainer so that you can stay safe in the weight room.

What is the typical way to pay a personal trainer? Weekly? Monthly? At each session?

Most personal trainers set up their own payment options for their clients. Many prefer to be paid at the beginning of the month. There are benefits to pre-paying: you solidify your "spot" so that it cannot be given away to someone else and it forces you to put your workout on your schedule as a priority.

Most trainers offer a discount to those who pre-pay for training packages. If you are only a "drop-in" client, working out with your trainer once a month or so, your trainer may have an option where you pay as you go. Each trainer is different.

Whenever you set up an appointment with a trainer it is important to respect that time. Come on time and be prepared to work hard. If you need to cancel, make sure you give your trainer 24-48 hours' notice or you may be charged for it.

When is a spotter needed for exercises?

A spotter is always needed when there is a good chance that the weight used is going to be too heavy. Many people that struggle with stability would benefit from having a spotter guide them through movements that require balance.

How does someone tone up in specific "problem areas"?

You can try and tone a problem area as much as you want but the fact is, if it is covered in a layer of fat, you will never see the effects of your hard work in the gym. If you want to tone up and lose fat in a specific area it will only happen through overall fat loss. This happens with diet and exercise. Never underestimate the power of a "clean" diet.—Think no sugars, no whites, no processed foods, no prepackaged meals, no fast foods etc.

Is it true that too much cardio can be unhealthy?

The statement, "too much of a good thing is bad" is true in this case. It is possible to do too much aerobic exercise. As with any exercise routine, it is important to take at least one day off a week to let your body rest and recover. There are definitely those people who get "addicted" to cardio and do it in excess of what is safe.

Being aware of the signs of overtraining can help you to know when a rest day is in order. Some of these signs are: irritability, perpetual soreness, fatigue, lack of enthusiasm for exercise, weight gain despite your excessive workouts, and a weakened immune system.

It is important to avoid doing the same cardio over and over without any variety. Always engaging in the same forms of cardio (such as running) will lead to a lot of wear and tear on specific joints. Vary your exercise choices and "cross train" as to avoid overuse of specific muscles and joints.

What are the benefits of hiring a personal trainer over just buying some DVDs that feature personal trainers?

When you hire a personal trainer, you have one-on-one attention and he/she will develop various workout programs specific to your needs, focusing on your respective goals. The trainer will motivate you, teach you proper form to keep you injury free and make your weak areas strong.

Exercise DVDs are a good alternative for those who might not be able to afford a personal trainer or who prefer to work out in the privacy of their own home. However a DVD is not "personal". The presenter on the DVD cannot see you and therefore cannot correct form if you are executing moves improperly.

If you are always using the same DVDs your body will quickly adapt to those exercises and you will stop seeing results. A good personal trainer will constantly change your exercise routines to create muscle confusion, which will help your body change and become stronger, faster.

Is it a good idea to walk or run with weights? Will this produce results more quickly?

This can be a controversial subject but it is never a good idea to walk or run with wrist or ankle weights strapped on. This will just create more stress on the elbow, shoulder, ankle, and knee joints.

If you are looking to burn more calories it would be safer to work out at a higher level of High Intensity Interval Training (HIIT).

If you really are set on the idea of running with extra weights, you can wear a weighted vest, which would allow the weight to be more evenly distributed without stressing the aforementioned joints.

—

Lisa Boucher, Owner and Personal Trainer
Train With Lisa
Saratoga Springs, Utah
801-368-7340 http://www.trainwithlisa.com
Lisa Boucher is a self-employed personal trainer in Utah, under the company name of Train With Lisa.

CHAPTER 5:

BODY4CHANGE

Founded in 2007, Body4Change was purchased by brothers Nick and Preston Rainey in 2011. Preston handles most of the business, leaving Nick in charge of all training programs.

Both brothers are very active and concerned with providing clients the best value for their money. The brothers feel human bodies are amazing things and they can help a client achieve the best body they can have.

What's the difference between "good carbs" and "bad carbs"?

"Good carbs" have other beneficial nutrients—fiber, vitamins, and phytonutrients. "Bad carbs" only provide you calories. These are often called "empty calories".

How does someone tone up and lose fat under their arms and around their triceps?

Use interval training or HIIT training to burn calories, then perform overhead tricep extensions. The benefit of putting your triceps over your head is that it puts the triceps in the best mechanical position to work. This position makes you stronger, which means more tone.

For people who are always tired, won't working out make them feel like they have even less energy?

If you're really tired and have a lot of stress there is no need to exhaust yourself at the gym. Start with a little and build from there. Once you're working out at the gym, listen to your body to know how much is enough. Don't listen before you go; it may tell you not to go. Once you're there, listen to your body. When your day is full of stress or you didn't sleep very much, you should perform exercises that are not heavy so you can do a lot of repetitions. Movement is energizing!

Is it true that stress makes people gain weight? What is the truth, if any, behind this?

Scientific research shows that not managing stress well causes an increase of a stress hormone called cortisol. This causes more visceral fat inside your abdomen, which is the really dangerous fat.

Fish seems to have a lot of fat in it. Will people gain weight if they eat too much fish?

You can gain weight eating too much of almost anything. However, you would need to eat a lot of fish to gain weight from that. A huge benefit of fish is the number of Omega-3 fatty acids. People need a 1:1 ratio of Omega-3 to Omega-6 fatty acids and most people have way more Omega-6 than Omega-3.

If someone is a heavy smoker, should their workout routine be adjusted at all? If so, how?

Yes and no. Yes, they will not be able to work out with the same intensity as a non-smoker. No, because everyone should need to get to a point where they are a little out of breath, back off, and then repeat that cycle frequently.

What are the biggest mistakes people make when hiring a personal trainer?

Not getting value! If the personal trainer is cheap, but they don't provide results then there is no value. If the personal trainer is super expensive, but the results are the same as if they hired another personal trainer that costs less, than they aren't getting the best value. Make sure you find someone who can and will spend time with you, gets results themselves, and has helped others achieve results similar to your goals.

What can people do to avoid back injuries when they're lifting weights?

There are 3 important ways to prevent back injuries while lifting weights.

1) Perform deep core exercises before you lift, but not to fatigue.

2) Use correct form. If you're not sure, find a personal trainer or physical therapy doctor that can help you.

3) Build slowly. Don't do 10 lbs. one day and 100 lbs. the next. If it feels like you shouldn't do it, then you probably shouldn't.

If someone eats very healthy, and they have an active lifestyle, do they still need to work out? Why or why not?

I always say that exercise covers up a lot of sins. Even if you're not "sinning" with what you eat you still need exercise for 2 important reasons. First, your heart needs practice pumping a lot of blood to help prevent cardiovascular disease. Second, by exercising all the muscles in your body you keep the neural circuits alive in your body, which improves your ability to balance and move. Both of those are crucial at all stages of life to prevent injury and pain.

Do minors typically need to get the permission of an adult or guardian, if they want to work with a personal trainer? If so, how does this work?

Minors need permission, but this is simple. All personal trainers have clients sign liability forms. The adult or guardian would just sign these for the minor.

Why do some people lift heavy weights while other people lift lighter amounts of weights?

Simple, some people know what they're doing and some do not. Everyone needs to attempt to lift heavy weight. However, heavy weight is relative. One major purpose of lifting weights is to improve the efficiency of our muscles. Increasing the weight we use increases the efficiency of our muscles.

Do personal trainers normally work with clients who are only free on weekends or during off-hours? What's typical in terms of when personal trainers are available?

Most personal trainers are flexible with clients' schedules. Many personal trainers schedule their personal lives during the day and plan to work in the evenings and on weekends because that is when their clients can train. If you have a personal trainer that won't work with your schedule find another one because, there is definitely one in your area that will work with your schedule.

If someone has back problems, or other physical limitations, how can they lift weights safely, without getting hurt?

Don't do anything that irritates your back! Often people have positions that alleviate and exacerbate their pain. It's crucial to lift weights in positions that alleviate the pain. Many physical limitations and pains are greatly improved through any type of movement.

What is the typical way to pay a personal trainer? Weekly? Monthly? At each session?

Monthly, or for a group of sessions are by far the most popular. The personal trainer will have a standard of how they normally do it, but if the client desires another way then the personal trainer is often flexible.

When is a spotter needed for exercises?

There are 2 scenarios when you need a spotter.
1.) If you are unfamiliar with the exercise and aren't 100% sure you are performing it correctly.
2.) If there is any chance that you may not be able to safely remove yourself from under the weight.

How does someone tone up in specific "problem areas"?

It's impossible to have 6-pack abs and flabby arms. Fat will leave all areas equally, and there is generally more fat in the problem areas. The key is to burn a lot of calories and increase your metabolism. This means you can't starve yourself every day. It's also essential that you exercise the "problem areas" in many different ways. This way you don't become the "skinny-fat" person.

Is it true that too much cardio can be unhealthy?

Theoretically, but it would take a lot of cardio. If it becomes an addiction or you are not eating and sleeping enough to recover from the amount of cardio you are performing, then it is too much. Our bodies are amazing. There are ultra-marathon races that are up to 100 miles that many people run in and are completely healthy.

What are the benefits of hiring a personal trainer over just buying some DVDs that feature personal trainers?

Most DVDs sit in a drawer or on a shelf. While not as beneficial as a live personal trainer, if someone will use a DVD daily they can be very beneficial. That being said, personal trainers provide a huge benefit over DVDs.

Personal plans are crucial for the client. Every client should know what the plan for them is 6 months and 12 months from now. DVDs don't provide this. The value of a personal trainer isn't in cool exercises, but in how they lead the progress of a client and ensure the client sees results.

Is it a good idea to walk or run with weights? Will this produce results more quickly?

Walk or run faster, or uphill. Weights cause you to change your mechanics and posture while you are walking or running. You should find an optimal posture that will help prevent increased pressure through joints which causes your body to ache.

—

Nick Rainey, Owner, Head Trainer
Body4Change, LLC
3210 N. Canyon Rd. #107,
Provo, UT 86404
801-427-8420
Body4Change@gmail.com www.Body4Change.com

CHAPTER 6:

SOCIAL WORKOUT STUDIO

Alice Raibon ran track in college and hasn't slowed down since. Besides keeping herself in shape for NPC Figure Competitions and working as a fitness model, Alice works her hardest for her clients. She will work with them at the gym or in-home, and listen with compassion and understanding of their needs. Her easy enthusiasm and knowledgeable workouts leave clients eager for their next workout, and loving their new lifestyle.

Is it true that stress makes people gain weight? What is the truth, if any, behind this?

Yes, stress makes people gain weight and most of the weight is in the stomach.

How does someone tone up and lose fat under their arms and around their triceps?

To tone up and lose the fat under your triceps you need to do strength training such as push-ups, triceps extensions, and triceps dips.

For people who are always tired, won't working out make them feel like they have even less energy?

No, working-out increases your energy level and gives your body a charge of energy.

What's the difference between "good carbs" and "bad carbs"?

"Good carbs", such as sweet potatoes and oatmeal, gives the body fuel and energy to be used throughout the day. "Bad carbs" slow the body down, as these carbs turn into sugar and fat in the bloodstream.

Fish seems to have a lot of fat in it. Will people gain weight if they eat too much fish?

Fish is high in protein and fatty acids, a good fat. It would take a great deal of fried fish for a person to gain weight from eating fish.

If someone is a heavy smoker, should their workout routine be adjusted at all? If so, how?

If you are a heavy smoker, yes your workout should be adjusted to low intensity cardio, and light weight training until you are able to do more.

What are the biggest mistakes people make when hiring a personal trainer?

The biggest mistake people make when hiring a personal trainer is getting one that's not compatible to them or their fitness goals.

What can people do to avoid back injuries when they're lifting weights?

To avoid back injuries you should wear a back brace to support your back. Use your legs when bending and keep your core tight.

If someone eats very healthy, and they have an active lifestyle, do they still need to work out? Why or why not?

Eating healthy and staying active does not mean you're flexible, that your body fat is low, or that you're fit.

Why do some people lift heavy weights while other people lift lighter amounts of weights?

Heavy weights are lifted by people who are trying to get bigger and stronger. Lighter weights are mainly used for toning.

Do personal trainers normally work with clients who are only free on weekends or during off-hours? What's typical in terms of when personal trainers are available?

Most trainers try to be available whenever the client is.

If someone has back problems, or other physical limitations, how can they lift weights safely, without getting hurt?

If you have a physical limitation you can still lift weights by doing light and seated weight training to avoid getting hurt.

What is the typical way to pay a personal trainer? Weekly? Monthly? At each session?

There is no typical way of paying your trainer, just work that out with your personal trainer before you begin.

When is a spotter needed for exercises?

A spotter is need when a person can no longer do exercises with weights through a full range of motion.

How does someone tone up in specific "problem areas"?

Isolations can help tone up certain areas but your body will tone all over, resulting in better health.

Is it true that too much cardio can be unhealthy?

Too much cardio ages the body and can cause joint problems.

What are the benefits of hiring a personal trainer over just buying some DVDs that feature personal trainers?

A personal trainer is better than the DVDs because a trainer will hold you accountable, motive you, educate you, and correct your form.

Is it a good idea to walk or run with weights? Will this produce results more quickly?

It is a good idea to walk or run with light weights only because it helps to burn fat faster. Though, it must be done properly to avoid joint damage.

—

Alice Raibon, Owner
Social Workout Studio
21141 Devonshire St.
Chatsworth, CA 91311
310-902-5387
www.workingoutwithalice.com

Social Workout Studio offers a range of services that can be used on a flexible schedule and budget. This is a fully-equipped studio where clients can schedule a personal one-on-one session with a trainer, or workout in small groups. Whether you are just getting started or looking for a more challenging workout, you will benefit highly.

CHAPTER 7:

FUNCTION 5 FITNESS

In this gym, the human body is the only machine you need. The personal trainers at Function 5 Fitness start with the fuel of that machine, assessing the caloric requirements of each client and establishing a proper diet for them. As clients implement these changes, the body is trained to live healthy, meeting the needs of the clients.

What should people look out for when hiring a personal trainer?

Make sure your trainer is certified by one of the top certifications and that their certification is current. It's perfectly ok to ask them what certification they have, and they should list them proudly on their bio or website. The Top 4 are: ACSM, ACE, NASM & NSCA but any certification they hold should at the very least be NCAA accredited.

Multiple certifications often mean that the trainer takes their education seriously and may have specialties. If you are special population or looking for a specific type of training, you may want to look into trainers that specialize. It's common for trainers to have additional certifications in strength & conditioning, corrective exercise, pre & post natal, nutrition or weight loss.

Just as important as credentials your trainer should be someone who understands your goals, doesn't impose their goals on you, and knows how to motivate you to achieve them. Make sure you meet your trainer in person for a trail session to see if you work well together.

If someone has a friend who is in good shape, who is willing to give them exercise advice, why is it still a good idea to hire a personal trainer?

Just because someone knows how to get their self in shape doesn't mean they are qualified to train others. Personal trainers have studied the human body, how to correct postural and muscle imbalances. They know how to coach, cue safe exercise form, know how to train and motivate a variety of different individual's needs and goals.

Is it true that people should take periods of time off from working out? If so, how long should these "workout vacations" last and how frequently should they occur?

My philosophy is that people should take time off rigorous workouts when life's pressures demand them to. We all know when those times are: breakups, family emergencies, injuries, a big work deadline, finals week, kids being sick, etc.

This doesn't mean that all activity must stop. I urge clients to keep up with corrective and recovery exercises like foam rolling, stretching, restorative yoga and walking when life has got them spun around. If clients have made fitness and health a priority in their life these hectic times shouldn't make up more than a week or so every 3 months. With a modest exercise program at all other times, this will still lead to good results and more importantly happier, less stressed out clients.

I think clients should pick 1-3 times a year when they ramp up their fitness for 3-6 weeks at time, when they know their life is not as hectic. I like to think of this type of fitness programming schedule as life-centered-periodization. It is practical and manageable with the modern life of most non-athletes.

What are some tips to help people stick with an exercise program and not quit?

First start off with a modest goal. For many people a goal of 3 days a week of working out is a good place to start. Once you have established this good habit you can add more days. Trying to bite off more than you can chew at first will set you up for failure and disappointment. You may be sore and need extra recovery in the beginning, which you won't get if you work out every day.

Second, pick something you actually like doing so that working out will be something you look forward to. My sport has always been Muay Thai, but when I retired as a pro athlete I found other sports and activities to keep me interested, workouts like tennis and Olympic weightlifting. If you take classes in a martial art, have a racquetball partner, compete in Roller Derby or love to surf you will be more likely to stay encouraged, active, and also meet health-minded people.

When you go to lift weight or run sprints (which are essentials for fitness) you will have a specific sport you are training to get better at, which improves your focus to the conditioning. Performance based goals always work better than body composition goals.

What is a "drop set"?

A drop set is when you perform a set of an exercise to failure (fatigue), but change a variable in a way that allows you to continue performing the set. For example, performing 10 push-ups from your toes, and then using an incline to immediately do another 5. Maybe doing 12 back squats at 145 lbs., then 5 at 125 lbs. right after. Drops sets can help with muscle hypertrophy (mass building).

If someone likes to listen to music, on a personal music player with headphones, when they workout, is this considered rude by most personal trainers?

It's important the trainer has the ability to communicate with you and give you cues on form, directions, and motivation.

Which types of people can benefit the most from a personal trainer?

Anyone can benefit, but the people who benefit the most are people that are committed to a fitness goal, open to learning, and changing their habits.

What are "boot camps" and why are they so popular?

Boot camps are large group fitness classes, usually held outdoors on in a big room like a rec center. Boot camp instructors are notoriously like drill sergeants, but some will let you know they have more of a cheerleader attitude to motivate clients. All boot camp attendees perform the same exercises, usually using body weight resistance or with minimal equipment like balls and bands. Boot camps often use circuit training as a structure.

Boot camps are best for those who already have some level of fitness knowledge, as you will not get much individual attention to your form. Some people also need a kinder, gentler approach to coaching and don't like feeling out of shape in a group setting.

How can people overcome junk food cravings?

Cravings are a possible sign of food addiction and metabolic issues. Most clients that come to me eat a diet that is too low in protein, too high in carbohydrates and sugar, and lacking in *quality* vegetables, fats and nutrients. With the Standard American Diet (SAD) of the USDA pyramid people will often get sugar/carb/processed food cravings, which have a poor structure for optimal health and a healthy metabolism.

To eliminate cravings I get people to stop eating processed food and start eating a real food diet with a good amount of protein, good fats, and nutrient dense veggies. This usually eliminates cravings in a couple of weeks. It's also important not to keep processed foods, snacks, or dessert foods in the house, as this can trigger cravings.

Do most personal trainers yell at people, like drill sergeants, to keep them motivated? What if someone wants to hire a personal trainer without being screamed at?

There are many types of trainers out there, and most are not drill sergeants. A good trainer will adapt their training style to their client's needs. I always try to find out how a potential client is best motivated so that I can place them with a trainer that suits their personality.

How does someone know if they're "over-training"?

Most people are not in danger of over-training unless they are professional athletes. However they are in danger of two things: under recovering and accelerating a program too fast.

The more you work out the more recovery you need. Recovery includes getting at least 7-9 hours of sleep every night, eating a healthy real food diet with attention to pre/post workout meals. Other recovery factors include foam rolling, massage, chiropractic adjustments, days-off training, down time, and smart supplementing with fish oil, BCAA's, vitamin D (if deficient) and herbal adaptogens. The more you train the more recovery you need, so be smart and don't overdo it if you can't afford to focus more on your recovery.

Accelerating a program too fast can cause the body to exhaust itself. Don't start from zero workouts to 6 a week right away. Ramp up slowly and increase intensity over time to get the best results.

If you are getting enough of the recovery listed above and have progressed your training in a smart manner, then you might be over-trained. Signs of over training include: insomnia, fatigue, lack interest in training, injuries, inability to recovery from injuries, and decreased performance.

How will a trainer know what program is right for their client?

They will ask questions about you and your goals and suggest a program based on their expertise. If you are not getting results with a trainer, schedule a time to reevaluate your program, goals, direction and troubleshoot alternatives. If the trainer doesn't think anything needs to change, but you are doing exactly what they say and not getting results, look for a new trainer.

Is it typically acceptable for people to bring their children to a personal training session?

Your trainer is not your baby sitter. Please get your childcare matters sorted out before scheduling a training session.

How much sleep should people get when they exercise regularly?

8-9 hours a night is best, 7 at the very least. Your body needs sleep to recover. You cannot lose body fat or build muscle without adequate rest.

Is it customary for a personal trainer to provide references of satisfied clients?

Please ask your trainer for references. If they are a legit trainer they will gladly give you a list of glowing testimonials of past and current clients.

What are some questions that people should ask a personal trainer before hiring them?

What certifications do you hold?
How long have you been training clients?
What do you expect of me?
What can I expect from you?
What is your cancellation policy (it's important to you are both clear on this)?
What happens if you have to cancel on me? (Some trainers offer a free session, some don't).
Do you offer a discount for cash payments (many do)?

Are there ways to reduce recovery time or soreness between workouts, without taking supplements?

Getting lots of sleep, 8-9 hours, and eating a real food diet free of processed foods helps recovery. Also foam rolling and massage are helpful.

What are some ways to verify the credentials/certifications of a personal trainer?

Most of the major personal training certifications have databases of current trainers who are certified with them. Simply go to the website and verify your trainer's certification once you find out which organization they are certified by.

Why don't crash diets work?

Crash diets stress out the body by limiting calories and/or certain macronutrients like fat or carbs. Crash diets may cause a decrease in weight for the short term, but often that is mostly loss of muscle mass and water weight that will come back when you start eating normally again. It's important to eat a balanced real food diet that fuels your workouts and fuels your fat loss so that you can lose fat gradually over time and keep it off.

I am much more concerned with fat loss than weight loss – it's important to make the distinction between the two. My clients get their body fat tested every 3 months with hydrostatic weighing to track results. This is the best method. You can learn more about it with a quick internet search to see if it's available in your area.

If someone feels that their trainer is pushing them too hard, or not hard enough how should they handle this?

First call or email the trainer and tell them you'd like to schedule a time to talk about your training. Communication is the key in any relationship and trainers can't read your mind! Tell them your concerns and see what they come up with to change your program or their training methods. If you don't like the changes and don't see any improvement, hire a new trainer.

—

Roxy Richardson, Trainer/Instructor
Function 5 Fitness
805 S. La Brea Ave
Los Angeles, CA 90036
323-272-4957 gym
323-934-0354 office http://www.function5fitness.com http://www.twitter.com/roxybalboa
https://www.facebook.com/MissRoxyBalboa

CHAPTER 8:

ELITE PERSONAL TRAINING STUDIO

Personal training, tandem training and group classes are all available at Elite. Starting with a free fitness assessment, most clients receive a nutrition plan and assistance in selecting the best trainer for their needs. After this, it becomes easy and fun to achieve fitness goals, with the staff at Elite cheering the client on.

If someone likes to listen to music, on a personal music player with headphones, when they workout, is this considered rude by most personal trainers?

If they're antisocial then they probably wouldn't want a *personal* trainer. If their trainer's that boring or that inept so the trainer doesn't use verbiage when training clients then they need to be fired. Not having music around is okay, but the trainer should be constantly talking to their clients. Rude? More like unimaginable and counterproductive.

What should people look out for when hiring a personal trainer?

When hiring a personal trainer for fitness people shouldn't have to "look out." People should only be aware of a few aspects. First, take advantage of the free session or sessions—always. If a trainer doesn't offer one, they're a joke. Since trainers should make a strong first impression, one session should be enough to know if you need to try a few more. Second, challenge the trainer, especially on that first day, by asking a lot of questions. If you don't have any questions—invent some.

Trainers are the versatile and knowledgeable health professionals and should conduct themselves as such in the fitness arena without even being prompted to be so. They should be all about the clients' physical needs. Change the questioning patterns with your trainer constantly and be a dynamic client so your trainer can respond. If they're truly knowledgeable about fitness and nutrition, they should know even more than they think they do!

Last—pricing. You determine the value of the trainer—not vice versa. You'll know you have a good trainer when you part ways with your money without breaking a sweat. The best trainers are truly undercharged for the services rendered. Trainers that wheel and deal with pricing are probably limited in their scope and knowledge. You won't see results past a couple weeks.

If someone has a friend who is in good shape, who is willing to give them exercise advice, why is it still a good idea to hire a personal trainer?

The first personal trainers were usually the buffest guys in the gym. People befriended them and learned from them. So can a friend be a good trainer? Absolutely. But, good shape doesn't mean they are good teachers, and being a trainer doesn't mean you are in good shape or a good teacher. A "trainer" should be both, a good teacher and in good shape.

A friend who is not certified can very well be a great trainer so there may not be a need to hire a trainer if this is the case, but this is rare. You trainer is different because they should have up-to-date knowledge, be super patient, be dependable, hold you accountable and have a genuine desire and ability to help, inspire, care, and motivate at all times. If this describes a friend, then they pretty much are a trainer.

Is it true that people should take periods of time off from working out? If so, how long should these "workout vacations" last and how frequently should they occur?

It depends on your goals and activities. If you pound your body in preparation for a competition or a race for weeks at a time, then you need probably twice as much recovery. This is for high-level athletes. If you are a moderate exerciser, just take one to two days off per week. If you do take time off from workouts, you should just maintain your gains and avoid detraining. So workout vacations can easily become quitting and that just doesn't work when fitness is a part of life.

What are some tips to help people stick with an exercise program and not quit?

You need to find dynamic, long term aspects that motivate you in your life. You can hang up clothes you want to fit into somewhere where you can see them each day, or leave fruit in the kitchen within eyeshot, or sign up for a competition, or plan an important event that you need to be fit for. Find a positive motivator rather than something vague like losing weight.

What is a "drop set"?

A drop set is a type of superset. You start with the heaviest weight you can lift for a few reps and lift to failure. Then drop the weights and pick up or get handed slightly lighter ones *immediately*. You should be able to do more reps than you did with the heavier weight, if you can't then you need a bigger variant between weights. Do this a few times and you have 1 drop set. It gives you a massive pump and allows you to potentially get better gains than regular training and saves time.

Which types of people can benefit the most from a personal trainer?

The question asked for who benefits the most; so out of everyone who doesn't workout 3-5 times per week, I would have to say overweight and obese men and woman ages 50+ would benefit the most. People over 50 tell me how much quickly their mobility declines as they age. Most people aren't done working (retired) by 50, so an immobilizing injury or a lifetime of bad posture can severely affect the way they live and work. This is a decline in quality of life that can be felt very, very quickly.

Around 50 seems to be an age range where people who are obese and overweight have the most health issues and can suffer sudden, fatal strokes and heart attacks. Combine these two facets and you have a pernicious recipe. Those who work out at least 30 minutes per day most days, on average, are known to live healthier and happier lives than people who don't.

What are "boot camps" and why are they so popular?

Boot Camps are classes that involve groups of people doing challenging exercises together. They're usually themed, affordable for clients, fun, engaging, and quick. Most people don't think they need trainers today (they do) and this is the best alternative. It is usually a fun and energizing environment but the trainers have to be fun and skilled in order for it to help the clients.

How can people overcome junk food cravings?

Cravings are not really just something you overcome, but there are ways to take your mind off of certain foods. Consider your goals, eating crap might damage your progress; consider your hydration because you might be more thirsty than hungry; think about how the food is made, if it makes you cringe, you don't want to eat it; keep snacks nearby so you can grab something else . . . almost anything is better than junk food pound for pound; drink water or eat something with fiber in it, this will stop the pangs for sweets and fill up your stomach; de-stress yourself with positive thoughts or another distraction and let the craving pass.

Do most personal trainers yell at people, like drill sergeants, to keep them motivated? What if someone wants to hire a personal trainer without being screamed at?

Drill sergeants yell to dissuade people from working hard so they can break them down and eliminate the "weak-minded." They want you to quit so they are left with the mentally tough. Training isn't about quitting, so yelling is negative and unhelpful. Trainers might yell on occasion, it's a way of getting attention or to increasing the positive energy of a class; but not for motivation.

If this bothers you explain it to them and they should stop yelling. Chances are if your trainer is aloof and power-hungry in the first session, they might be bad trainers. If your trainer screams constantly at you, especially if you are noticeably jilted, they're on a power trip and they don't want to help you, only themselves. Fire them.

How does someone know if they're "over-training"?

Over-training leads to mostly, it seems to me, mental fatigue. Your body, especially in those who are constantly training, can train and work way, way longer than you probably even will ever know. Humans are designed to survive physical stress and this means if you have to keep moving for days without stopping, your body will surprise you.

Over-training is relative because we are all different genetically and fitness-wise. However, when your nervous system and brain has had enough, it will shut your body down to survive. Over-trained people will have trouble doing the mentally – not physically – taxing activities of life. They will have trouble eating, sleeping, reading, concentrating, speaking, overall focus, and will probably have some type of chronic pain and be stressed. They will appear hyper and aloof. Over-trained individuals will be, for example, those who don't eat more than once a day but are scatter-brained and workout twice a day or more in combination.

How will a trainer know what program is right for their client?

Trainers assess their clients in the first few sessions to see what type of program will fit. Good trainers have access to hundreds of program styles to modify. Trainers ask, constantly, about their clients' feelings on their workouts. If the fit is wrong, the trainer adjusts first. The best way to know if the program is right is really to ask the client.

The clients monitor themselves closely, and the trainer monitors the client from a different perspective. If the results are positive, that means the assessment was correct and the exercise prescription was beneficial.

The trainer is a fitness professional and must be knowledgeable in exercise prescription; if they're not, they would not be certified. This really should not be trial-and-error. It is based on experience and knowledge and rapport.

Is it typically acceptable for people to bring their children to a personal training session?

Children of a certain age can benefit by watching their parents and even engaging in the exercises as long as their parents are focused. Children that are too young really should be in daycare or away from the area of training. They could get hurt which will definitely distract the parent and reduce the quality of the workout session.

How much sleep should people get when they exercise regularly?

Less than 5, maybe 6, hours is too little and you will be stressed out the next day. If you're stressed, your workouts will suffer and your body won't be able to get into better shape. More than 6.5 hours is safe. Rest helps your body recover and remove byproducts of exercise and nutrition. If you interrupt this necessary bodily function for weeks, your body will adjust and slow down its metabolism, so you won't perform at average levels.

Is it customary for a personal trainer to provide references of satisfied clients?

Good trainers have testimonials. Newer trainers won't but that doesn't mean they are horrible trainers. So it's not customary, but good trainers have strong rapport with former clients and can use them as references to help newer clients make the right decision.

What are some questions that people should ask a personal trainer before hiring them?

How often should I train with you and how often without you there? How should I be eating? What can I expect in 1 month? 3 months? 9 months? Have long have you been training? Are you certified? What's your contact info? How often to you work out? Do you have more clients? How should we keep track of my progress? Where is the water fountain? How fast can I expect results/final result? What's your specialty/scope/style of training? How can I stay motivated?

Are there ways to reduce recovery time or soreness between workouts, without taking supplements?

Assuming the "supplements" in the question are sports supplements and food supplements, not really. Stretching and using foam rollers help to reduce the feeling of being sore, but if you're sore, it's only because of muscle trauma and your body just needs time to repair. Soreness is a result of muscles being broken down because they are not used to the eccentric movement of workouts, and that happens when you train hard or are not used to training.

What are some ways to verify the credentials/certifications of a personal trainer?

You can call the accrediting organization and ask. You can online to the organization and type in the trainers ID, after the trainer gives it to you. The best way is to contact the company by phone and have them look up the trainer. If it's a degree ask the trainer to see their diploma.

Why don't crash diets work?

There's a reason way there are so many crash diets marketed in America. They do work, if you want to lose a lot of weight in the short term (like

1-3 weeks), and then gain it all back. In the long-term, they are useless. Considering most clients want a long-term habitual lifestyle change from their trainer, this is a moot point for trainers.

Clients consider crash dieting sometimes. They cannot learn to live without one of three macronutrients for the rest of their lives, which are often what crash diets limit. So it's impossible to crash diet and actually keep weight off for more than a few months. I have yet to hear, see, read about, or talk to *anyone* who has crash dieted and permanently lost weight.

Mostly crash dieting fails because it never becomes a habit; it's just a painstaking shortcut that no one can sustain. Pseudo-intellectuals that advise people to crash diet are sad excuses for health professionals and are probably profiteering from ill-advised people.

Changing habits is simply the only way to lose weight and crash diets are not habitual. They reduce the calories you eat but do so by restricting some foods you might need, with the promise of grandiose too-good-to-be-true results that keep you wanting to achieve them. It is the same story every time unfortunately, and reducing calories works no matter what foods you eat and what time of day you eat them.

If someone feels that their trainer is pushing them too hard, or not hard enough how should they handle this?

Firstly, use your words. Say "this is easy", or "I don't feel this" or repeatedly say "what's next". If they don't get the idea, you might have a crappy trainer teaching you. Conversely "I'm afraid of hurting myself with heavy weight", "I'm taking a break" or "hold on" should break the tempo of an overly difficult workout.

Secondly, tell your trainer what you want specifically, very specifically, so they understand that what they are doing needs adjustment, such as "I only want to work legs today." Clients only say these things if they are looking for control or if the trainer is distancing themselves from the client.

Third, attempt the hard work out and only do a couple reps. A good trainer knows how to adjust this to make the client work harder at their near-max or max. If it's too easy, do the exercise super-fast or talk a lot while lifting, no good trainer lets this happen for too long. You could then try to tell them outright, as this is a business the trainer should be giving you a great product.

Say/ask, "This is too easy/hard, I want to feel the best workout possible please, can you give me a new exercise/weights?" Last, your trainer should pretty much know how to assess your exertion levels constantly, some by sight or speech alone. If they're not responsive to you, they need to improve or get fired.

—

Johann Francis, Trainer /Instructor, C.S.C.S.
Elite Personal Training Studio
1068 Park Avenue
San Jose, CA 95126
www.elitesj.com

Elite was founded by Laura Swain in October of 2008. Laura's goal was to help people lead healthier, happier lives regardless of their financial status or fitness level. Elite was the first functional training space in the Willow Glen area of San Jose, which means using bodyweight exercises and free weights instead of machines. This effective fitness model has become incredibly popular over the last 5 years-and Elite is proud to be one of the pioneers of the functional training movement in San Jose.

CHAPTER 9:

TOTAL FITNESS AND HEALTH

Chris Abbott opened Total Fitness and Health to share the joy of a healthier, stronger life. Perseverance and persistence have allowed Chris to compete in Ironman competitions, triathlons, and work with people as diverse as their goals. Chris loves to meet new people and educate them on health matters.

If someone has a friend who is in good shape, who is willing to give them exercise advice, why is it still a good idea to hire a personal trainer?

It's always best to seek the advice of a professional because they know what's best for you. A friend may know of a really cool and effective workout for himself but that same workout may not be the best solution for anybody else. Form is the key factor in getting maximal results without risking injury; it takes a trained professional's eye to catch compensations and know when to regress or progress an exercise.

What should people look out for when hiring a personal trainer?

Does the trainer perform some sort of movement screen prior to the first workout and does he/she have the knowledge to give you a workout that doesn't involve machines? Also are they themselves fit?

Is it true that people should take periods of time off from working out? If so, how long should these "workout vacations" last and how frequently should they occur?

In the event that someone has been pushing too hard for too long a "workout vacation" will actually do the person a world of good. Depending on how over-trained the person is, a week to a week and a half is sufficient to recover from a long period of over-training. Planned periods of over-training are completely different and typically the "workout vacation" is not really a vacation but different workout of lighter intensity compared to the previous weeks. A properly planned training program should prevent a client from having to take an unnecessary "workout vacation".

What are some tips to help people stick with an exercise program and not quit?

Start off very simple and very easy to build confidence and motivation. People need to have the feeling of success early and often when starting a new training program. Running new clients through a gauntlet of exercises only to leave them crippled the next day is no way to start an exercise program. Start with the basic movements and master those first.

Note that simple and easy doesn't mean the client sees results right away, the key is learning to do the things that matter perfectly at first, then push up the intensity.

What is a "drop set"?

When a person works out at a weight then removes a fraction of the weight and performs another set.

If someone likes to listen to music, on a personal music player with headphones, when they workout, is this considered rude by most personal trainers?

While I don't promote it, I do have some clients that like the listen to headphones during their workout. As long as they can hear me that's all that matters. Personally I don't feel a lot of trainers think it's rude.

Which types of people can benefit the most from a personal trainer?

Everyone can benefit, no matter what age or gender. Unfortunately, society has become such that people as young as 17 years old are developing back issues linked almost directly to their lack of exercise and mobility. A proper strength program is good for anyone who falls in that category, all the way to senior citizens who have limited mobility due to age.

What are "boot camps" and why are they so popular?

Boot camps are organized group workouts. The term boot camp often gives the impression of a hellish class or environment. While some fitness instructors make it their goal to provide such a service, there are more that provide great quality in terms of effectiveness and low risk of injury. They're often much cheaper than normal one-on-one training or even semi-private training. These group settings also help to create a community environment which can help people feel they are not alone in working towards a goal.

How can people overcome junk food cravings?

Eat more protein. Protein signals the release of hormones that literally tell the body you're full. Oftentimes snacks and meals full of carbs with little to no protein will enable someone to eat massive amounts yet still be craving something sweet. If after a high protein and vegetable meal you're still craving something sweet, have a piece of dark chocolate; it won't do any harm to your nutrition and it'll satisfy your craving.

Do most personal trainers yell at people, like drill sergeants, to keep them motivated? What if someone wants to hire a personal trainer without being screamed at?

I've seen my fair share of personal trainers in different settings and I would have to say more often than not, people are not being yelled at by their trainers. If it's a concern, the client simply needs to interview different trainers. Do some research online, go in for a trial session, and narrow down trainers until you find one. Most trainers give at least 1 session to a potential client for free.

How does someone know if they're "over-training"?

Oftentimes they'll see one or a variety of these symptoms: a decrease in performance, sleeplessness, irritability, loss of appetite, constant aches and pains, and or the onset of illness due to weakened immune system.

How will a trainer know what program is right for their client?

Proper assessment techniques consider: nutritional habits, lifestyle habits, what the person does for a living, what types of movements are required on a daily basis, some sort of movement screening to show any potential red flags or areas of concern, and detailed, specific goals from the individual. Every bit of information counts when creating the proper program for someone.

Is it typically acceptable for people to bring their children to a personal training session?

No, unless they're older than 17 and the client has previously spoke to their trainer about bringing them in. Otherwise, it becomes a distraction for the trainer and the client.

Is it customary for a personal trainer to provide references of satisfied clients?

Not customary, but I feel it definitely helps from a business perspective, as well as helping the client. When they're able to read a few testimonials from previous and or current clients, new clients will feel more comfortable in training with you.

What are some questions that people should ask a personal trainer before hiring them?

Anything and everything related toward their fitness goal. If the trainer is good and knowledgeable, they should be able to answer anything related to getting that person the best results possible.

Are there ways to reduce recovery time or soreness between workouts, without taking supplements?

Yes, massages help. If that's not an option a cheaper and more readily available option is the use of a foam roller. If that still doesn't help, a 5–7 minute ice bath to relieve soreness.

What are some ways to verify the credentials/certifications of a personal trainer?

Don't bother looking for what certification a trainer has, as they're all just about the same and don't say much about the trainer. Ask the trainer what types of things they do to continue their fitness education. Seminars and other certifications outside of basic personal training will indicate they truly value the service they provide to clients. Most trainers are willing to reinvest in themselves in the form of seminars, mentorships, or extended certifications.

Why don't crash diets work?

Often they're too drastic and only provide temporary success, if any. Once the person reverts back to their old ways the weight goes back on. Building a foundation of healthy nutritional habits is a much longer method but one that yields greater result for life.

If someone feels that their trainer is pushing them too hard, or not hard enough how should they handle this?

Clients should tell the trainer exactly how they feel. While trainers may seem to know a lot about their clients, ultimately the client will know more about themselves. If the client feels something is too much, or not enough, they should be comfortable talking about it with their trainer. If they don't feel comfortable then maybe they should find another trainer, a good relationship with their trainer is key.

—

Chris Abbott, President/Coach
Total Fitness and Health
11611 San Vicente Blvd. Suit 100
Los Angeles CA 90049
518-332-7636
Chris.Abbott@TotalFitnessandHealth.net
www.Totalfitnessandhealth.net

Whether its weight loss, building lean muscle, sports performance, or rehabilitation, I've helped someone like you reach a goal just like yours. My semi-private training model allows you to share the cost of a 1-on1 personal training session with one other person. You, (and potentially one other person) work with me at the same time. Each of you performs your individual training program. Scheduling sessions is easy with my online scheduler; simply search for your desired appointment and book online. Clients just like you get results in a matter of weeks. Don't waste time, get fit now!

CHAPTER 10:

BLUNT FORCE TRAINING

Not only is Tiffany Coolidge ranked as one of the top 10 trainers in Denver, she recently won the Editor's Choice Award for best trainer in 5280's Top of the Town 2013. What's more, she won her first boxing match by TKO and she sat on the board of directors for the Women's Campaign School at Yale University. She's also been featured in The Denver Post.

Tiffany Coolidge is more interested in health than the socializing of a big box gym. When she founded Blunt Force Training, it was a no-frills gym that makes the best of personal ability to constantly improve a healthy lifestyle. She believes that working out is not a social event, which makes the connections forged between people that much more meaningful.

What are some tips to help people stick with an exercise program and not quit?

Unfortunately, there aren't any tips or tricks. It's hard work. Changing your lifestyle is never easy, but committing to fitness gets easier if you make it a habit or routine. Celebrate small milestones and accomplishments, i.e. running your first mile, increasing weight in your first lift, even making it to the gym when you almost went back to bed. Try to set a goal other than weight loss, such as running your first 5K, so it's not just about a number on the scale.

What should people look for when hiring a personal trainer?

Look for a trainer who shares your vision and helps you reach your goals. Know if you are going to be more comfortable with a male or female and what your motivational style is, i.e. drill sergeant, screamer, or more mellow. Also, make sure they know any injuries or health conditions before your first workout. If a trainer doesn't do an initial consultation with you before your first workout, that should be a red flag.

If someone has a friend who is in good shape, who is willing to give them exercise advice, why is it still a good idea to hire a personal trainer?

You want to make sure you find a certified trainer who puts safety and form first. For example, the wrong motion or lift with too much weight could create lifelong injuries. Your friend's fitness goals, metabolism, health history and body are likely different than yours, while a certified trainer works with a variety of clients and has experience to work with all levels of physicality.

Is it true that people should take periods of time off from working out? If so, how long should these "workout vacations" last and how frequently should they occur?

You always want to give your muscles proper time to heal and recover. Try not to train more than 3 days in row without an off day, as your body's ability to repair muscle will be lessened. Always listen to your body, if after a new or challenging workout you feel extra sore the next day, take it as a rest day and come back stronger for the next workout.

What is a "drop set"?

Drop sets are when you lift weight with the highest weight you can for set, i.e. 15 lbs. on shoulder press, then you continue cutting the weight down 12 lbs., 10 lbs., 8 lbs. until your muscle fatigue and you cannot complete any more reps.

If someone likes to listen to music, on a personal music player with headphones, when they workout, is this considered rude by most personal trainers?

Not unless it's during a personal training session where it's important for the client to be able to hear instruction on proper form. During independent workouts, music has been shown to lessen perceived levels of exhaustion and is a great motivator.

Which types of people can benefit the most from a personal trainer?

Everyone! Personal trainers do the research for new and unique exercises so you don't have to. Some people may go to the gym on their own five days a week and get caught in the same boring workout routine and plateau. They don't have someone pushing them to improve session after session and creating muscle confusion for optimal results.

It's very easy to perform lifts and moves with bad form and create compensations and instabilities in your muscles, weakening your body over time. Good personal trainers emphasize form and proper alignment at all times to avoid this.

What are "boot camps" and why are they so popular?

Boot camps are group training sessions. These can grow as large as you're willing to tolerate. Some people are motivated and thrive on the energy of others. You don't get the personal attention of one-on-one trainings, but there should be a balance of group and individual attention, to make sure you're doing the exercises correctly. Most boot camps are high energy calorie burners that many people crave.

How can people overcome junk food cravings?

Remember what you're working toward. It's a healthy lifestyle, not a healthy meal or single choice. Reward yourself for milestones and not pebbles. Try to find substitutions for what you are craving. If it is sugar, reach for some fresh fruit, for salt or potato chips, try some baked kale chips for a similar taste without the fat and calories.

Do most personal trainers yell at people, like drill sergeants, to keep them motivated? What if someone wants to hire a personal trainer without being screamed at?

It really comes down to compatibility. Find a trainer that knows how to motivate you. Some of my clients respond well to positive encouragement, some are inwardly motivated, and some need a series of small goals.

How does someone know if they're "over-training"?

When tired muscles turn into pulled muscles. When they are training more than 3 days in a row without a rest or recovery day, or when they feel completely run down.

How will a trainer know what program is right for their client?

The client and the trainer need to be on the same page to identify a training routine that matches that client's unique and individual goals.

Is it typically acceptable for people to bring their children to a personal training session?

It can be a challenge, but as long as the client can focus on his/her workout and not the child, then exposing their kids to a healthy lifestyle is a good move. It also depends on that club or fitness center's rules.

How much sleep should people get when they exercise regularly?

As much as they can! Sleep is key to the muscle's recovery and growth. 7-9 hours is optimal.

Is it customary for a personal trainer to provide references of satisfied clients?

A good trainer should always have references ready and available for prospective clients. The references should be from a variety of clients, including male/female, of different ages. Individuals who have achieved their goals are best, such as post pregnancy, ran first marathon, post injury, etc.

What are some questions that people should ask a personal trainer before hiring them?

What are your specialties? What kind of certifications do you have? What is your training style? When can I expect to see measurable results?

Are there ways to reduce recovery time or soreness between workouts, without taking supplements?

Your muscles and body work hard during a workout, so you need to supply them with protein and amino acids for recovery. Obviously, all-natural clean foods that are high in both protein and amino acids are preferred, lean fish, chicken, beef, quinoa, leafy greens, etc. Ice baths immediately post workout also work quickly to reduce inflammation, along with an Epson salt hot bath before the next workout.

What are some ways to verify the credentials/certifications of a personal trainer?

Ask to see the certification from the trainer or verify with his/her association that accredited them. ISSA, NASM, ACE are some of the bigger programs, but there are a variety of other small programs and schooling.

Why don't crash diets work?

Crash diets are aptly named because they happen quickly and you have to repair the damage at some point. Many of these diets starve your body and can alter your hormone levels and your metabolism. Once the diet fails, it's difficult to stabilize your hormones and jumpstart your metabolism again.

Unfortunately, after a crash diet, things get worse before they get better, which can be frustrating for people. Sometimes they actually gain weight as their body transitions to a healthier lifestyle. The fact is a healthy diet coupled with a robust fitness regimen is the best way to lose weight and feel great. You want to move from "diet" to healthy lifestyle.

If someone feels that their trainer is pushing them too hard, or not hard enough, how should they handle this?

Again, you'll need to be on the same page as your trainer. S/he should know your fitness goals exactly and if you're not being pushed enough or too much, you may need to revise those goals with your trainer.

—

Tiffany Coolidge, Owner
Blunt Force Training
2031 Bryant St.
Denver, CO, 80211
(303) 324-9500
Tiffany@blunt-force.com
www.blunt-force.com

Blunt Force Training is a 9,000 square-foot training facility that specializes in total body strength and conditioning with a focus on cardio and core. Blunt Force also specializes in training fighters in MMA, Jujitsu, and Boxing. It is located next to Sports Authority Field and is minutes from downtown.

CHAPTER 11:

JOHN FERNANDEZ

Bringing the latest in research and technology to his work, John Fernandez works the brain just as well as any other muscle. Instead of telling a client what to do or what to eat, John explains why he thinks these are good ideas for the client. As an athlete, John knows how the body works as a whole unit and finds a way to improve the overall functionality.

Is it true that people should take periods of time off from working out? If so, how long should these "workout vacations" last and how frequently should they occur?

Life is mobility. Exercise may not be the most important aspect of life to most individuals but it is the vehicle that carries what is important. To make real progress one must do strength training sessions with all-out effort for 3 days a week, and cardio-respiratory exercise in-between. One day off is only recommended to preserve your enthusiasm and motivation to exercise.

Your blood carries all the nourishment you cells need to live up to their full capacity. When circulating, blood nourishes your body but also carries away waste product. The real benefits of exercise come with years of sustained movement with purpose.

Did you know that at rest only 20% of your blood flows through your muscles? In a fit individual, that percentage rises, and with exercise that percentage rises to 80%.

What should people look out for when hiring a personal trainer?

Finding the right personal trainer can be one of the most important decisions in life. Hiring a personal trainer isn't like buying a packaged product. What you get, and more importantly the results you get are based on the experience and skills of that personal trainer.

When trainers work with people to change their bodies, they're also working with them to change their minds by learning new habits. In regards to exercise these things aren't taught in exercise physiology class, they're acquired through the trainer actually being an athlete with hands-on experience. How can a personal trainer identify with the energy and stress demands he is imposing on another's skeletal, muscle and cardio-respiratory system if he has not experienced it himself in every aspect possible?

One of the greatest assets of a personal trainer who is an avid athlete is that they have a better understanding of the human body during movement. This invaluable experience allows them to structure a safe yet effective training program and, in some cases, diet. I say, "some cases" because some personal trainers while doing well with athletes, will struggle to help weight loss and general fitness clients because they simply can't relate. As athletes they've always been in shape and don't understand the difficulties a general fitness client may be facing.

So finding a trainer who is an athlete themselves with experience is certainly an attribute one should look for when hiring a trainer.

One should also seek a trainer who has made personal training their passion and profession, not their let-me-stay-busy-job. There are many students with basic personal training or nutritionist credentials or none at all, working while attending school or working in an industry outside of fitness. Many may have no passion for fitness, while some with a passion for fitness feel working with clients isn't their "calling". These trainers are often in school or working for other things, which makes them unconsciously not committed to the client's needs.

It's hard to find good quality fitness professionals. They may meet the qualifications on paper, but those qualifications have to come to life. The practical application is the challenge.

Some may have years of experience and knowledge, may be organized and know how to manage their time, have a good work ethic, etc., and they can say a lot in regards to the science of the human movement system. However, the issue isn't just finding a personal trainer with great credentials. It's finding the right personal trainer in an industry in which is just emerging.

And because the industry is still in its infantile stages it will be awhile before the supply of fitness professionals equals the demand. Right now, the demand for a personal trainer with qualifications and experience is higher than the supply, so often an unqualified trainer fills that spot.

If someone has a friend who is in good shape, who is willing to give them exercise advice, why is it still a good idea to hire a personal trainer?

People don't reach their desired results simply because they do the wrong exercises at home or in the gym. They don't reach their desired goals because they lack structure and fail to tap into their true potential. Aside from giving your day more structure, being motivated and given clear direction, a personal trainer corrects your bad habits, posture and technique, all which allow you to perform better.

A good personal trainer also knows how to scale down, or up, the intensity of an exercise session without necessarily having to decrease or increase the load of the weight. This is where personal trainer excels in value. Stop exercising and start training!

What are some tips to help people stick with an exercise program and not quit?

Most people join health clubs or hire trainers for fitness, but they stay for fun and results. Sociability is a major key for many health club members and personal training clients. Find a gym or health club that compliments your lifestyle and hire a trainer who can not only educate but can also prescribe exercises that mimic your exercise personality. Trainers should keep changing up your routine to keep you engaged and challenged.

What is a "drop set"?

A drop set is the simple technique where you perform a set of any exercise to failure or just short of failure, then drop some weight and continue for more repetitions with the reduced poundage.

Even though you may reach a point of momentary muscular failure after 8-12 reps in a conventional straight set, you haven't reached absolute failure, you've only reached failure with that poundage.

In a single straight set performed to failure, you don't activate every fiber in a muscle group. You only recruit the number of fibers necessary to lift a particular weight for the desired number of repetitions. By stripping off weight and continuing the set, you cumulatively recruit more and more "reserve" muscle fibers.

Drop sets hit the "stubborn" muscle fibers "deep down," causing growth that normally couldn't be achieved by stopping after a single set of six to twelve.

Bodybuilders love drop sets because they're concerned purely with cosmetic improvements and not athletic performance. That's why bodybuilders prefer drop sets—because they're decidedly geared towards increasing muscle size (hypertrophy).

By contrast, you don't see a lot of football players, sprinters or other athletes using drop sets, because drop sets are not conducive to strength, power or speed gains. In fact, most athletes want strength and power without bulk, so drop sets are usually nixed. However, if pure muscle is what you desire than drop sets are ideal.

If someone likes to listen to music, on a personal music player with headphones, when they workout, is this considered rude by most personal trainers?

Actually it's a fact that listening to music during exercise will increase your endurance by 15%. However, if you have a positive and motivational relationship with your trainer you won't find a need to block him and the environment out. Besides, if you have reached the point in which you can perform a set without the coaching and cues from your personal trainer than he has done his job and you should/need to move on. Tuning out your trainer while executing a set defeats the very reason why you have hired a trainer in the first place; getting instructions.

Which types of people can benefit the most from a personal trainer?

The types of people that eat and breathe and want to maintain their functionality. The type of people who want to live and not just exist, especially when he or she is over 50 years of age.

A good program has universal scalability and personal trainers make it a perfect application for any committed individual, regardless of their experience. Personal training is for everyone but more so for those who sit during their commute to and from work, who sit at work and think they get enough exercise going up and down the stairs, for those who lack the motivation to go to the gym, and for those who go to the gym but lack the motivation to push harder.

—

John Fernandez, Owner
Personal Training
San Mateo, CA
415-351-8124
http://www.personaltrainingsf.com

John Fernandez is a fitness competitor and avid athlete who has followed the science of exercise and has been training for over 20 years, incorporating his vast knowledge of nutrition, exercise, and sports-specific training towards his own goals and achievements.

John's program delivers a fitness that is, by design, broad, general, and inclusive. His specialty is not specializing. Healthy living requires that we push, pull, run, throw, climb, lift, jump, and decelerate movement effectively and safely regardless of whether or not you play athletics. Athletics is a specialized pursuit. John's goal is to support the specialist, but reward the generalist.

CHAPTER 12:

SCOOP PILATES AND

PERSONAL TRAINING

Husband and wife team Phillip and Tracey Griffin combined their twenty years of experience in creating Scoop Pilates and Personal Training. From prenatal Pilates, to Krav Maga and Breast Cancer recovery fitness, Scoop Pilates offers something for every point in life. The studio is a combination of spiritual retreat and energizing innovations, all designed to let clients find their healthy lifestyle.

What is a "drop set"?

A drop set is designed to fatigue a muscle within by doing as many reps as possible, until you can't do anymore and you drop the weight. Start with, for example, cable bicep curls with 70 lbs. Repeat the curl until you can't do another rep, then immediately lower the weight to 50 lbs. Do the cable bicep curls with 50 lbs. until you have to drop to 30 lbs.

What should people look out for when hiring a personal trainer?

People should look to see if the trainer is certified and what type of certification, or certifications, they have. Is it a credible certification or something they got online by paying a fee? Is the trainer designing a program based on your goals and needs, and not their comfort level? For instance, you want to train for a triathlon, but they're having you do strength training to put on muscle and look good. A trainer should also be in decent shape. They don't necessarily have to have 3% body fat or be able to run a marathon, but they should be able to practice what they preach.

If someone has a friend who is in good shape, who is willing to give them exercise advice, why is it still a good idea to hire a personal trainer?

The friend may be able to train themselves, but you may have a different body type, different nutrition or cardio requirements. Suppose that person tells you to run 3 days a week because it works for them, but you have bad knees or hate running. There are so many other types of cardio you can do, but your friend won't know about those exercises. Advice does not always fit everyone.

Is it true that people should take periods of time off from working out? If so, how long should these "workout vacations" last and how frequently should they occur?

It really comes down to listening to your body. If you work out regularly 3-5 times a week you may reach a point where you feel run down, mentally or physically. In that case take a few days off, or even a week if you need it. Sometimes, though, instead of taking a "vacation" you should just scale back your workout.

For example, if you're used to lifting heavy weights then lift lighter weights, or incorporate more bodyweight exercises to your routine for the next week. Or if you're used to running 25-35 miles a week scale it back to 10-15 miles or do more swimming or biking for a while.

What are some tips to help people stick with an exercise program and not quit?

Go into a routine knowing that at some point you may feel like quitting, but when you get to that point keep pushing through. Give yourself a day or two, but that's it. Get right back to it. Go back to the goals you had when you started your program. Find your motivation. Something motivated you to start a program in the first place. Whether it's your kids, spouse, or just you, remember that when you feel like quitting.

If someone likes to listen to music, on a personal music player with headphones, when they workout, is this considered rude by most personal trainers?

I think most trainers do consider this rude, but if it's what the client wants then they can. I would tell them to have the music low enough that they can hear my instructions.

Which types of people can benefit the most from a personal trainer?

If you're new to working out, or just not sure of what to do when it comes to exercise then definitely look into a personal trainer. But really, anyone can benefit from a personal trainer. Even professional athletes have personal trainers. Personal trainers are there to help you to the next level, regardless of what level you are currently on.

What are "boot camps" and why are they so popular?

Boot camps are group classes designed to build strength and endurance through a set of interval style workouts. The exercises are a mixture of strength, endurance, and agility. Most boot camps are designed to have more military-style exercises, such as push-ups, jumping jacks, running up hills, etc. They are popular because they are challenging in nature. The group setting provides a sense of camaraderie, and people motivate and push each other.

How can people overcome junk food cravings?

Try to find healthy alternatives. Try to eat baked chips instead of regular chips, a fruit bowl instead of cookies, sugar-free Jell-O, etc. If you look long enough you will find something you like.

Do most personal trainers yell at people, like drill sergeants, to keep them motivated? What if someone wants to hire a personal trainer without being screamed at?

I've rarely come across trainers who yell at their clients. Sometimes with certain clients you may have to raise your voice to give them a little extra push, but yelling like the trainers on the *Biggest Loser* is not common. If you have a trainer who yells like that but don't want them to, let them know you don't respond to that type of training. You're the client! If they won't change, get a different trainer.

How does someone know if they're "over-training"?

If you're getting to the point where you don't have energy, or where your body is not recovering, this is a good indicator of overtraining. When you get to that point, take a couple of days off or scale back your workouts until you get re-charged.

How will a trainer know what program is right for their client?

Determining a client's needs should come from their training and experience. The program should be based on their goals, medical conditions, exercise history (what's worked or hasn't worked for them in the past), availability, and their nutritional habits.

Is it typically acceptable for people to bring their children to a personal training session?

It's not typical that people bring their children to a session. Sometimes it's just unavoidable and you make do. As long as it doesn't become routine, or interrupt the session it should be fine.

How much sleep should people get when they exercise regularly?

Ideally, you want to get 8 hours, but sometimes that's not realistic for people. I tell my clients to try for 8 but get a minimum of 6.

Is it customary for a personal trainer to provide references of satisfied clients?

Not in my experience. Most people have already done a little research on the trainer before they decide to become a client.

What are some questions that people should ask a personal trainer before hiring them?

Are you certified? If so, what are the names of the certificates and certifying agency? What are your specialties (ex. rehab, training athletes, training elderly, etc.)? How much experience do you have? Are you dependable? Are you punctual? You'd be surprised how many trainers aren't.

Are there ways to reduce recovery time or soreness between workouts, without taking supplements?

Ice helps. Stretching and/or massages will help as well. Also, a good diet can help. Getting the adequate amount of carbs, proteins, and fats will help with muscle recovery, bone and joints, and inflammation. Eating a good post-workout meal to refill the nutrients lost from a workout also helps with recovery.

What are some ways to verify the credentials/certifications of a personal trainer?

You can ask the trainer. Most trainers will have their certifications visible to everyone.

Why don't crash diets work?

Crash diets are hard to sustain. Most of them will leave you without adequate nutrients over the long haul. Try to get on a diet that you can follow for the rest of your life. I tell my clients to try and live by the 80/20 rule. 80% of the time, try to eat healthy and the other 20% of the time eat whatever you want.

If someone feels that their trainer is pushing them too hard, or not hard enough, how should they handle this?

They really need to communicate this to their trainer. I've seen many times where a client will go to another trainer and say their trainer was too hard or too easy, instead of communicating this to their trainer. A good, professional trainer will not be offended, but instead make the necessary adjustments.

—

Phillip and Tracey Griffin, Owner and Instructor/Personal Trainer
Scoop Pilates and Personal Training
8817 Highway 6, Suite 470
Missouri City, TX 77459
281-778-6801   info@scooppilateshouston.com   www.scooppilateshouston.com
Scoop Pilates and Personal Training was opened in May of 2010 in Missouri City, TX. We offer mat and reformer Pilates classes in group or private settings. We also offer 30 min. and 60 min. personal training sessions. We design programs specifically for the client, which includes advice on nutrition and cardio routines.

CHAPTER 13:
JAYE ELIZABETH HARRIS TRAINING

By combining nutrition, physicality, emotional balance and spirituality, the human body can become a work of art through science. Beth Harris works to match her activities to her clients' needs, even using webcams for remote training. You can find many examples of her clients' success stories on her website at www.jayeelizabethharris.com.

What's the difference between "good carbs" and "bad carbs"?

"Good carbs" get absorbed slowly into our systems, avoiding spikes in blood sugar levels. Avoid bad carbs by eating fewer refined and processed carbohydrates, which are absorbed quickly and cause spikes in blood sugar levels.

How does someone tone up and lose fat under their arms and around their triceps?

Fat loss is an overall metabolic process of depleting fat stored. Women tend to carry fat around their triceps to a greater extent than men. The best plan is a healthy diet, and a balance exercise program including cardio and strength training.

For people who are always tired, won't working out make them feel like they have even less energy?

When you don't exercise and have poor eating habits your metabolism will slow down. Healthy individuals tweaking their diets get an immediate increase in energy and improved sleep state. Starting an exercise program may make you a little more tired initially, within the first week, but in reality it has the opposite effect. Drastically improving energy levels, concentration, memory, improving sleep, the list goes on.

Is it true that stress makes people gain weight? What is the truth, if any, behind this?

Yes, stress can make you gain weight. Everything is stress; good stress and bad stress. Good or eustress is things like exercise that is good for you. Bad stress or distress is losing your job or wrecking your car, or just being overworked. When we encounter stress, our bodies begin to adapt and repair, then return to baseline. But what happens if we don't return to baseline? If we continuously live in a state of constant repair and *distress?* We are perpetuating catabolic, or breaking down, processes within the body.

Cortisol, known as the "stress hormone" is secreted during times of physical or psychological stress which can alter and disrupt normal secretion. This promotes weight gain but also affects where you store fat on your body. Research shows excess altered cortisol release can cause fat deposition in the abdominal area rather than in the hips.

Fish seems to have a lot of fat in it. Will people gain weight if they eat too much fish?

Not all fish has a lot of fat. Tilapia only has one gram of fat per ounce. Many fish are full of omega-3's which help reduce inflammation, stabilize moods, reduce asthma, and keep your heart healthy. If you eat too much of anything you'll gain weight, and your diet should be appropriately portioned with carbs, fat, and protein.

If someone is a heavy smoker, should their workout routine be adjusted at all? If so, how?

Our blood cells, the little transporters of our bodies, have an affinity for carbon dioxide. If you smoke, the carbon dioxide inhaled is absorbed better, taking all the seats on the bus so the oxygen cannot get to where it needs to go. Heavy smokers will have a disadvantage when it comes to breathing in general, and a program would have to be modified accordingly.

Is there any truth to the claim that exercise can help improve brain function and/or mental focus? If yes, how?

Exercise is the best medicine! Exercise improves functioning of all body systems, helping to regulate hormones and increasing the rate of oxygen getting to your cells.

What are the biggest mistakes people make when hiring a personal trainer?

Assuming because they are "certified" they are qualified. Currently personal trainers are not regulated by the government, so anyone, and I mean anyone can claim the title. Find a trainer who has not only a certification approved by the NCCA, but an educational background in exercise science. Experience with people of a similar health situation as you will be important in selecting a trainer.

What can people do to avoid back injuries when they're lifting weights?

Always keep good form. Follow a program appropriate for your level of fitness and expertise. Your program should strengthen your functionally and prepare you for the activities of daily living.

If someone eats very healthy, and they have an active lifestyle, do they still need to work out? Why or why not?

Active lifestyle is a very loose term. The American College of Sports Medicine recommends 3-5 days of cardiovascular exercise for 20-60 minutes at 60-90% heart rate max, 2-3 days of strength training, 2-4 sets targeting all major muscle groups, and 2-3 days of stretching targeting all major muscle groups. These recommendations are set forth based on solid research and studies determining what behaviors result in health benefit.

Do minors typically need to get the permission of an adult or guardian, if they want to work with a personal trainer? If so, how does this work?

Minors are not considered adults because they are not ready to make adult decisions. Deciding on an individual to assist you changing your life and health outcomes is a huge decision not to be taken lightly.

Why do some people lift heavy weights while other people lift lighter amounts of weights?

It's all about specificity. Lifting lighter weight for more reps targets muscular endurance, lower reps and higher weight/strength targets power.

Do personal trainers normally work with clients who are only free on weekends or during off-hours? What's typical in terms of when personal trainers are available?

All trainers are different. Personally my schedule is very flexible.

If someone has back problems, or other physical limitations, how can they lift weights safely, without getting hurt?

Only work with trainers with experience and education in working with injured people.

What is the typical way to pay a personal trainer? Weekly? Monthly? At each session?

Sometimes monthly, sometimes by session, it often depends on if you are hiring through a gym or not. Remember if you are going to a gym and hiring a trainer, the gym takes a percentage of the fee and determines the parameters of programs offered.

When is a spotter needed for exercises?

In my opinion it's better safe than sorry, but always when you're hitting your limits. Personally anything above 75% max.

How does someone tone up in specific "problem areas"?

Never should anyone workout simply to target problem areas. Your body is composed of trillions of cells all working towards the same purpose, why would you only train one area? Only working your chest, for example, will eventually make your chest stronger than your back which will result in injury. It's important to understand human movement and know you don't want things off balance.

Is it true that too much cardio can be unhealthy?

Your heart is a muscle too, don't overdo it! Balance is key.

What are the benefits of hiring a personal trainer over just buying some DVDs that feature personal trainers?

Do you really learn anything about yourself in those videos? How to eat, when, what, how to exercise, what works best for your body type and metabolism?

Is it a good idea to walk or run with weights? Will this produce results more quickly?

Walking with weights is a way to add intensity to your workout. Remember you only want to modify one component at a time: intensity, time, duration, mode, frequency. If you are walking 30 minutes and decide it's getting too easy, you don't want to add weights and increase time at the same time. How quickly you reach your goals is a reflection of many variables, and can't be determined by walking with weights or not.

—

Beth Harris, Owner and Personal Trainer
Jaye Elizabeth Harris Training
386-303-1574 http://www.jayeelizabethharris.com/
Beth Harris is a mother, athlete, Health & Fitness Pro, nutritional consultant, motivator, writer, fitness model and figure competitor. She holds a B.S. in Exercise Science from FSU, and certifications with the National Strength and Conditioning Association (NSCA)-Certified Strength & Conditioning Specialist (CSCS), American College of Sports Medicine-Health and Fitness Specialist (HFS), and American Council on Exercise-Certified Health Coach.

MOVING FORWARD

Congratulations on making it to the end of this book! We hope that you realize and appreciate the immense level of real world knowledge that you've just acquired. The one thing you may be feeling at this point is a bit of "information overload", due to the many tips, pieces of advice, and strategies that are jammed into this book.

If you are feeling a bit overwhelmed from everything you've just learned, allow us to offer you one final piece of advice: Take a day to let your brain absorb all of the information you just learned. As they say: "Sleep on it". If you attempt to try and remember and implement everything you just learned, your efforts may tend to be scattered and a bit unorganized. Instead, take a day off from the information. If you do this, you're likely to find that you develop a sense of clarity and a better perspective on the information.

Once you've taken a day to allow yourself to re-focus in this way, we encourage you to slowly go back through the book, writing down the actionable information that you intend to implement. Simply reading and understanding the information is not enough. By writing down the information that you plan on implementing, it will allow you to put a clear plan of action into place for yourself.

As you go through the information, don't worry about the order in which you write things down. The first thing to do is to just get the information down on paper. There are many great strategies and tips within this book, but the goal here is for you to extract the exact advice that you will be taking action on. Don't worry if you are unsure about whether or not you will be taking immediate action on certain advice. Just write down everything that you may possibly take action on.

Once you've compiled this list of action steps and "maybe action steps", begin to prioritize this list. In other words, re-write the list with the actions that you know you're going to take at the top of the list and the action items that you may not take action on towards the bottom of the list. By organizing your list in this way, you will be able to build a practical, useable to-do list, from the information you learned in this book. Once you've done this, you will be in an excellent position to start taking focused steps, with clarity and purpose.

As we mentioned at the beginning of this book, most peddlers or fitness products and information hope that you keep buying their stuff. In keeping with the rebellious nature of this book, we encourage you to stop buying more fitness stuff and start implementing what you just learned in this book! Just as we have shared interviews with real world experts who actually do what they talk about in this book, it is our hope that you, as the reader, will take real world action on the information you've learned here.

Wishing you all the best in your action-taking, fitness and nutrition endeavors!

ABOUT PROMINENCE PUBLISHING

Prominence Publishing is a niche book publisher, specializing in helping small business owners separate themselves from their competition.

We publish and distribute non-fiction books. We are pleased to work with a wide range of authors to bring specialized titles to market. We produce single-authored books as well as compilations books, like this one.

Have you always wanted to write a book? We can help you.

We do not take a generic approach to book publishing. While there are certain "best practices" within the industry, we evaluate each title on a case-by-case basis, to determine the most sensible strategy.

We view the relationships that we have with our authors as partnerships. This unique approach in our industry ensures that all parties are "on the same page", when it comes to the direction of each project. While our industry experience has allowed us to develop effective strategies, we are always open to hearing fresh perspectives and ideas. We view the authors with whom we work, as valuable individuals who have key insights. We believe that this philosophy of cooperation and communication with each author, is one of our greatest strengths.

To learn more about our services and our company, we invite you to contact us at www.ProminencePublishing.com.

www.ingramcontent.com/pod-product-compliance
Lightning Source LLC
Chambersburg PA
CBHW060424290526

45791CB00002B/868